HOW TO SLEEP LIKE A CORPSE

7 WAYS TO PASS OUT IN 120 SECONDS

BENJAMIN TAYLOR

CONTENTS

INTRODUCTION

Sleep is a finite resource that a lot of people tend to take for granted. These days, it's so easy to get swept up in the hysteria and pandemonium of hustle culture. Of course, that isn't to say that it's bad to work hard. In fact, it's great if you find a way to maximize your potential by applying yourself in ways that allow you to excel. That's a mark of a life well lived. However, in an age where so many people flaunt their achievements and milestones on social media, it can be so easy to get overwhelmed. The competitive fire in us gets stoked and we push ourselves to work just as long and hard as the next guy. What we don't realize is that allowing ourselves to get swept up in such a manner is dangerously bad for our health. And when it comes to devoting more time to working hard, you have to realize that you're also taking time away from something else. Do you know what people often cut out of their schedule in order to make time for work? Sleep.

Again, in a world where people are desperate to succeed and make names for themselves, there seems to be very little talk about the value of sleep. There are so many gurus out there who preach about productivity and making the most out of your time through discipline and habit formation. I'm one of those people. But it's just as important that we dedicate much of our global rhetoric to talking about the value of sleep and the role that it plays in our lives. Sleeping is not just some activity that you do whenever you're tired. It's so much more than that. There is a literal science to sleep that not many people have taken the time to understand or appreciate. There is a reason why sleeping is such a vital activity for human beings. Unfortunately, many of us seem to take sleep for granted, and that's what this book is trying to address.

Many of you who are reading this now might actually already be experiencing some trouble with falling asleep at night. It's either that or you're just generally curious about the kind of impact that sleep can have on your life. Ultimately, not too many people will pay attention to the way that they sleep unless they start feeling the negative effects of it. You may notice that your days are moving just a little slower because you didn't get a good night's sleep the night before. You may have people telling you that you woke up on the wrong side of the bed consistently because of how irritable and unnerving you are. You may have difficulty focusing or getting things done because you feel so tired all of the time. All of the things that have been mentioned so far are symptoms of certain sleeping conditions you may be going through.

Sleeping problems are much more common than you may think. It's just that not a lot of people take the time to really look into the science of sleep and how it works. For them, sleep is a natural involuntary act that the body goes through every single day. By reading this book, you are separating yourself from these people. You don't see sleep as some chore that you need to fulfill every day. By reading this book, you are actively choosing to pay closer attention to the way that you sleep so that you will be in a better position to reap the benefits from it. You are also actively choosing to confront the problem surrounding your sleeping habits so that it will no longer serve as a hindrance to you pursuing your dreams and achieving your goals.

There's nothing to be ashamed about if you have issues with sleeping. Again, it's a fairly common condition. Remember that the first step to solving any kind of problem is admitting that there is one. It's only when you acknowledge that you need help with solving your sleeping woes that you are able to actually start getting better. In this book, we will go over why it's a good thing that you're paying attention to your sleep patterns. We will be discussing why sleep is important and how bad sleeping habits could compromise your quality of life. Then, we are going to go over what the possible causes and factors are contributing to your sleeping problems. We are also going to go over some basic habits, routines, and exercises that you can practice in order to counteract your symptoms. This book will also delve deeper into the science of sleeping along with all its facets, such as sleeping position, environmental design, and habit formation. Ultimately, we will talk about everything that you need to know as you get started on your journey to achieving better sleep at night.

By the time you finish reading this book, you should have the foundational tools and knowledge that you need to improve your sleeping habits. You should also have a more well-rounded perspective on the science of sleep and how you can approach your sleep problems methodically. And most importantly, reading this book should help you foster a healthier and more wholesome relationship with sleeping as a whole.

CAUSE AND CONSEQUENCE

The first step to addressing any problem is understanding why the problem exists in the first place. You may be eager to learn all about all of the secrets and hacks to getting a good night's sleep. Waking up feeling energized and refreshed every morning is finally within your grasp, and you just can't wait. However, before we can get to the actual hacks and solutions to help you get better sleep, we need to take the time to address the causes of your sleep difficulties to begin with. It doesn't matter how many helpful hacks and tips you employ to try to improve the quality of your sleep. If you're still engaging in bad habits that will compromise the quality of your sleep, then it all gets canceled out.

Aside from that, we are going to talk about the consequences of not having good sleeping habits. To do this, we need to have a deep and fundamental understanding of the role that sleep plays in our lives. Why do human beings need to sleep anyway? What happens in our bodies while we sleep? What's the worst thing that could happen if we don't employ proper sleeping habits for the rest of our lives? Before you can hack the concept of sleeping, you need to develop a better understanding of what the activity entails and the many nuances to the sleep process.

Again, you might already be eager to get the practical advice that will lead to you getting better sleep. However, it wouldn't be sustainable for you to just do all of the practical activities without understanding why they're important. This is why you need to understand the theoretical aspects of sleep science so that you are in a better position to apply all of the practical advice in your life after that. Sleep really is one of the most important aspects of a person's day, and many of us take it for granted. The goal of this chapter is to completely revitalize your perception of sleep and the role that it plays in shaping your life.

WHAT IS SLEEP DEPRIVATION?

To put it simply enough, sleep deprivation simply means not getting enough sleep throughout the course of a typical day. Most experts typically recommend that adults get around seven to eight hours of sleep every night for optimal health (Blaivas et al., 2020). Sleeping for any less than the recommended amount classifies as sleep deprivation. Not many people take the idea of sleep deprivation seriously. However, this could lead to some health problems and complications.

Sleep deprivation can come as a result of a variety of different possible factors. In the next phases of this chapter, we will go deeper into the causes of sleep deprivation and what happens to your body when you're constantly not getting enough sleep.

WHAT ARE THE CAUSES OF SLEEP DEPRIVATION?

As mentioned previously, there are many possible factors that could contribute to sleep deprivation. Some of them are the result of voluntary behavior, like if you constantly go out partying or are fond of hanging out with friends late into the night. Sometimes, it's because you have a working schedule that has you awake during odd hours. Other times, you might have certain medical or biological conditions that keep you from getting quality sleep at night. There are also a lot of people who struggle to go to sleep because of certain emotional or mental health issues like anxiety or depression.

When it comes to behavioral choices, a common reason people don't get enough sleep is because they feel like they don't have enough hours within a day to do everything that they want. So, they try to cram as many activities as possible within a 24-hour time period. However, doing so many things can often come at the expense of devoting an ample amount of time to sleep. Instead of going to sleep at your proper bedtime, you might be reading books, browsing through social media, talking to friends, or watching TV. These are conscious choices that people make which prevent them from going to sleep at the appropriate hour.

As far as medical issues are concerned, there are many conditions that could either impair or compromise the quality of one's sleep. Two common conditions associated with disruptive sleep are sleep apnea and snoring. Usually, people who have sleep apnea are those who have problems with their respiratory tracts. They might have sinusitis, which prevents them from taking in the appropriate amount of oxygen through their nose. Other people might have deviated septums, which can impair their breathing. Whatever the case, not taking in enough oxygen during sleep can impair one's ability to get into a deep sleep (which is a stage of sleeping that we can talk about further in later chapters). Another medical condition that could contribute to sleep deprivation is thyroid disease. It is known that having an overactive thyroid gland can cause sleep problems because it triggers an overstimulation of the nervous system. Essentially, the condition has your brain firing up even at night when you're supposed to be winding down. Aside from the physical complications, other people also struggle with certain mental health conditions that keep them from getting enough sleep at night. It's not rare for people who have depression or anxiety to struggle with insomnia. A lot of getting quality sleep at night has to do with mastery over the mind. If the mind is too cluttered or hyperactive, getting a good night's sleep can be almost impossible.

Sleep can also be disrupted by a person's medicinal or dietary intake. There are certain maintenance medications that people take frequently which could potentially lead to sleep deprivation. For example, medications that are used to treat attention deficit hyperactivity disorder are known to disrupt a person's natural sleep cycle. A person's food and drink intake can also dramatically impact the quality of their sleep. One popular culprit that leads to sleep deprivation is caffeine. Having either too much caffeine or taking it too late within the day can lead to sleep deprivation at night.

Of course, there are also environmental factors that need to be taken into consideration, such as temperature, noise, ambient light, and others. If a room is far too cold or too warm, it may cause difficulties in getting enough sleep. If there's too much noise within a sleeping environment (such as when there's a crying newborn in the bedroom), that can disrupt a person's sleep. If a person is exposed to too much blue light at night, their mind may be tricked into thinking that it's not supposed to be shutting down for sleep yet. We will learn more about these environmental factors and how you can manipulate them to promote better sleep in a later chapter.

Ultimately, going to sleep at night isn't just a matter of shutting your eyes and hoping that you'll eventually drift off into a sleeping state. It's so much more complicated than that. As you may now realize, various conscious choices that you make during the day contribute to whether you get a good night's sleep later in the night.

WHAT HAPPENS WHEN YOU DON'T GET ENOUGH SLEEP?

Think back to the last time you spent most of the night in bed tossing and turning while waiting for yourself to fall asleep. If this is a fairly common occurrence for you, then you might be familiar with the feeling of not getting enough sleep. You don't always feel at your best the next day. You're either cranky, irritable, tired, unmotivated, or a combination of all of those things. However, what you may not realize is that these aren't the only effects of sleep deprivation. If you consistently don't get enough sleep at night, it could affect your quality of life on a more fundamental and serious level. Both your physical and mental health are put at risk if you consistently engage in poor sleeping habits. In this segment of the chapter, we will cover the many ways that sleep deprivation can negatively affect your life.

Compromised Cognitive Function

While you're sleeping, your brain is busy forming certain connections that are designed to help you process any information or data that you've acquired while you were awake. However, if you don't sleep properly, it could impair your brain's ability to process this data and help you form memories. Aside from that, not getting enough sleep can impair your overall cognitive function that is required for you to do deep and meaningful work. It can kill your focus, creativity, and logic. It will be much harder for you to get through tasks if you are sleep deprived. This is why it's not ideal for students to stay up late the night before an exam. It could do much more harm than good.

Mood Swings

Moodiness and irritability are also common effects of sleep deprivation. This is mostly because of the hormonal imbalances that take place in your body as a result of not getting enough sleep. The volatile nature of your hormones can make you much more emotional and hot-tempered than usual. At first, your mood swings can be just that—simple manifestations of emotional aggression here and there. However, if left unchecked, these emotional imbalances could potentially escalate to more serious mental and emotional conditions like anxiety or depression.

Weakened Immune System

Your immune system is an amazing product of evolutionary biology. The human body is continuously evolving as it finds ways to immunize itself against any harmful bacteria or diseases that could compromise your overall health. However, if you're not getting enough sleep, then your ability to fight off these diseases will be compromised. Sleep deprivation results in the weakening of your immune system, which could lead to you becoming more susceptible to viruses. As a result, you're more likely to get sick more often when you consistently don't get enough sleep.

Poor Motor Function and Reflexes

If you are a professional athlete or just someone who likes to maintain a relatively active lifestyle, then you know how difficult it can be to engage in any kind of demanding physical activity when you don't get enough sleep. On an episode of *The Tim Ferriss Show* podcast, NBA superstar LeBron James revealed that he makes it a point to always get at least eight to 10 hours of sleep every night. James is notorious for maintaining a very strict health and wellness regimen, and sleep science plays a huge part in that. James even admitted to sometimes sleeping for as much as 12 hours. The legendary basketball athlete is of the belief that getting a good night's sleep is crucial to finding success on the court.

Conversely, if you happen to have poor sleeping habits, then it could compromise your athletic performance. At best, you walk a little slower or you might bump into a few things here and there because your body is just a little fogged up. At worst, you could get into a serious accident like failing to make a proper turn when you're driving your car. Poor sleep can also lead to compromised coordination. This means that you become more susceptible to tripping or folding your ankle while you're walking.

Increased Risk for High Blood Pressure, Diabetes, and Heart Disease

Unfortunately, not getting enough sleep does much more damage than just impairing your cognitive function and motor abilities. It doesn't just make you feel more irritable or compromise your immune system. It could also potentially lead to more serious medical conditions like high blood pressure, diabetes, and heart disease.

Usually, when you don't get enough sleep at night, you might notice that your heart is acting a little hyperactive throughout the following day. This is typically because sleep deprivation can lead to increased blood pressure. Whenever you have high blood pressure, it can result in inflammation of various parts of your body, especially within your circulatory system. Naturally, this kind of abnormality within your circulatory system can cause too much stress on your heart, which could potentially lead to some kind of cardiac disease.

Aside from that, not getting enough sleep is also linked to diabetes. This is because a lack of sleep actually impacts your body's ability to release insulin. This is a very important hormone that helps regulate your body's blood sugar levels. If you have a compromised insulin release, then that means there might be too much blood coursing through your body. Having high blood sugar can also lead to medical complications like heart disease and kidney failure.

Weight Gain

Another effect of sleep deprivation is weight gain. When you eat, it often takes a while for your stomach to send the appropriate signals to your brain that you've had enough food. However, when you lack sleep, these signals might get a little muddied or they can take longer to reach your brain. This means that you may end up eating more than you really need, which could potentially lead to a caloric surplus. This kind of consistent overindulgence in food will lead to weight gain, and as you may already know, factor into the development of other diseases like diabetes and heart disease.

Lower Sex Drive

Sleep experts are of the opinion that not getting enough sleep at night can result in lower libidos for both men and women (Peri, 2010). This means that regardless of your gender, you are likely to have a lowered interest in sex if you're not getting enough sleep. A lot of this has to do with the fact that not getting enough sleep can lead to feeling tired, sleepy, and tense. All of these factors contribute to you the unlikelihood of you getting into the mood for sex. Physiologically speaking, not getting enough sex might not be that big of a deal. However, if you're in an intimate romantic relationship with someone, then not getting enough sex could negatively affect the quality of that relationship.

UNDERSTANDING THE SCIENCE OF SLEEP

When it comes to understanding *why* human beings need sleep, there is no definitive answer yet. Many scientists and experts over the years have given valid explanations over what happens in the body when you sleep and why sleep is good for you. However, there is no single explanation for why people need sleep at all. It's mostly a combination of many different factors that could lead to the improvement of one's overall quality of life.

In the past, it was believed that sleep was an innately *inactive* activity. Scientists used to think that falling asleep merely meant falling into a deep state of physical and mental inactivity. However, research over the years has shown the opposite. All throughout a typical sleep cycle, both your mind and body go through various processes that are designed to promote optimal health and wellness. When you go to sleep at night, you go through a series of cycles which are made up of different sleep stages. Each stage of sleep serves a specific function that affects your body in a different way. Ultimately, your sleep cycles are segregated into two distinct phases: REM (rapid eye movement) and non-REM sleep.

As you're beginning to fall into the sleep cycle, you start off in non-REM sleep. This particular phase is composed of three distinct stages. The first stage of non-REM sleep is when you're still awake and you're consciously trying to fall asleep. The second stage is when you're already in what is called *light sleep*. During this stage, your heart rate and breathing will slow down just a little while your body temperature drops. Also, at this stage, it's still relatively easy for you to get woken up by light, movement, or noise. The third stage of non-REM sleep is dubbed as *deep sleep*. During deep sleep, your body's heart rate and breathing slow down significantly. Your body remains completely still, and it's much harder for you to get woken up while in this stage. It's during this phase of sleep that is most crucial for your mind's ability to process and retain information. Aside from that, deep sleep is when your body is hard at work when it comes to repairing muscles, organs, and other cells. It's also during this stage when your body is boosting its immune system. So, getting enough deep sleep is a crucial aspect of promoting physical health and wellness.

Then there is the REM phase of your sleep cycle. During the REM phase, your brain activity will gradually start to pick itself up again. Your eyes will also be moving about even as they remain closed (hence the name). This is also typically the stage of sleep wherein you experience vivid dreams. While you're in REM, your body also goes into a state of atonia wherein your muscles are temporarily paralyzed, except for your eyes and muscles necessary for breathing.

REM sleep is also a phase of sleep that is crucial for the cognitive development of your brain.

The amount of time that you spend in each stage of the sleep cycle can determine the overall quality of your sleep. Ideally, this is what a typical sleep cycle should look like:

Stage 1: Awake = one to five minutes

Stage 2: Light Sleep = 10 to 60 minutes

Stage 3: Deep Sleep = 20 to 40 minutes

Stage 4: REM = 10 to 60 minutes

A typical night of sleep should be made up of around four to six sleep cycles. The length of a standard sleep cycle can vary from person to person. In fact, not all sleep cycles that you have in one night will be uniform in length. However, sleep cycles typically last for an average of about 90 minutes. Now, you might be asking yourself why it's important for you to learn about these sleep stages in the first place. Well, you need to understand that not all forms of sleep are created equal. Taking a 30-minute nap in the middle of the day isn't necessarily going to make up for having missed 30 minutes of deep sleep the night prior. This is why it really pays to have a sleep tracking device such as a smartwatch that can help you determine the quality of your sleep. Remember that it's not just about how much sleep you're getting. It's as much about quality as quantity.

When it comes to inducing a state of sleepiness, there are two things that you need to pay attention to in your body: your circadian rhythm and your sleep drive. Think of your circadian rhythm as your body's natural clock. It's what's in charge of letting your body know whenever it's time to be awake or to sleep. Your circadian rhythm is a big factor when it comes to influencing your body's ability to fall asleep soundly or not. Your circadian rhythm is also greatly influenced by various environmental and behavioral factors. For example, whenever your body is sensing a lot of blue light from the sun or harsh LED lights, this signals to your circadian rhythm that it's supposed to be awake. This is why it can be difficult to fall asleep at night in a brightly lit room. Your circadian rhythm can also be impacted by the food that you eat. It's known that alcohol and caffeine can disrupt your body clock and therefore compromise the quality of your sleep.

Aside from the circadian rhythm, you also need to familiarize yourself with your sleep drive. Think of your sleep drive as your body's ability to crave sleep. It is to sleep what your appetite is to hunger. The greater your appetite, the easier it will be for you to eat more food. The higher your sleep drive, the easier it will be for you to get more sleep. Your sleep drive functions similarly to your hunger signals in a lot of ways. If you go for too long without eating, your body is going to constantly send signals to your brain that it needs food. It's the same with sleep. The longer you go without getting quality sleep, the stronger the signals are for your brain to seek proper sleep. However, there is one major difference between sleep and hunger. Ultimately, you have control over whether to satiate your hunger or not. It's not like your body will involuntarily make itself full on its own. On the other hand, if you go long enough without getting any sleep, your body will slowly shut itself down on you as if forcing you to sleep. You might have experienced this before when you're in the middle of a meeting or when you're commuting on the train. Your body is running on fumes because of how tired you are and it decides to just fall asleep against your will. The only factor that can influence your sleep drive is how long you can go without falling asleep.

FINAL THOUGHTS

As you may have discovered over the course of this chapter, sleeping is much more nuanced than most people realize. There are actually many factors that can influence one's quality of sleep. Also, the act of sleeping in itself is more than just lying down and shutting your eyes for a few hours every night. Vital processes that are important for your health, wellness, and overall productivity take place all throughout your body while you sleep. As we make our way through this book, we will learn more about how we can manipulate certain factors in our lives so as to make sure that we improve the quality of our sleep every night.

4-7-8 BREATHING METHOD

*I*n the previous chapter, we learned all about the many factors that can contribute to sleep deprivation at night. A lot of the time, people have difficulty falling asleep as the result of hyperstimulation within the mind. This stimulation can be caused by anxiety, overthinking, and general mental agitation. The 4-7-8 breathing technique that we will discuss in this chapter is designed to counteract the hyperactivity that's taking place in the mind so as to induce a sense of relaxation. It's a fairly simple breathing technique that was developed by Dr. Andrew Weil, and it has principles that are rooted in *pranayama* yoga.

We will be talking about what this technique is, why it works, and how you can perform it properly to help you fall asleep at night. Many people who regularly practice the 4-7-8 breathing technique every night before sleeping have found that it allows them to more seamlessly drift into a state of sleep.

WHY DOES IT WORK?

To reiterate, we've already established that mental activity and stimulation is a huge impediment to falling asleep at night. The more stimulated your brain is, the more difficult it will be for you to drift into a sleep state. So, as a way to counteract that overstimulation, scientists and experts have recommended breathing techniques. In yoga and meditation, breathing is typically used as a tool to promote relaxation and calmness. While this activity may seem completely arbitrary, it's actually founded on many principles that are rooted in science. Whenever you stay mindful of your breathing, you are promoting the better distribution of oxygen throughout your body. Try to think back to a time when you were stuck in a stressful or tense situation. Did you find yourself experiencing shortness of breath? This is your body's natural response to stress and anxiety. When you're lying awake at night, your mind may be running at 100 miles an hour as it's trying to process different concepts and ideas that may be bringing you stress. Focusing on your breathing will allow you to relieve some of that pressure and stress, thereby calming your mind and putting it in a state that is more conducive for sleep.

When you force your mind to consciously think about your breathing, it distracts from all of the things that are causing you to have stress and worry. Aside from that, you are bringing more oxygen to your cells, which can help induce a state of relaxation and calm. In the words of Dr. Weil, engaging in mindful breathing functions somewhat like a natural tranquilizer for your nervous system. Of course, there are many other breathing techniques and frameworks out there that are rooted in the same principles. However,

Dr. Weil's 4-7-8 technique seems to be the most popular, especially among the sleep science community.

If you're just starting out with this exercise, it's possible that your mind can drift in and out of mindfulness over your breathing and that's okay. Over time, with enough repetition, you will gain better control over your mind as if it were a muscle. Many proponents of the 4-7-8 breathing technique say that the effects of the exercise become more potent with every practice.

HOW DO YOU DO IT PROPERLY?

The first thing that you need to do whenever you want to practice the 4-7-8 breathing technique is to find a place wherein you can sit or lie down comfortably. Even though the 4-7-8 exercise is mostly effective for inducing a state of drowsiness, it's also a practice that you can employ at random points of the day whenever you feel overwhelmed or stressed.

You can prepare for the exercise by resting the tip of your tongue against the roof of your mouth just behind your front teeth. Your tongue should stay in this place throughout the entire course of the exercise. This may require a lot of mindful effort at first, but you will find that it will become second nature to you over time. So, don't feel too stressed about struggling with it for the first time.

Open your lips slightly and expel any air in your body through your mouth. Make sighing or whooshing sounds if you can. Close your lips and inhale silently through your nose. Try to count to four in your head and let your inhale last throughout that entire duration. After the initial four seconds, hold your breath and count to seven. Conclude the breath by gradually expelling all the air from your body through your mouth for the duration of eight seconds.

Repeat the process as many times as necessary. Typically, you only need four full breath cycles in order to feel the effects of relaxation and calmness. Keep in mind that whenever you're practicing this technique, the phase wherein you hold your breath is the most important part. It's also recommended that you do not practice this technique in situations or environments wherein you should be on full alert, such as when you're driving a car. Again, this is a practice that can help you fall asleep more easily, but it doesn't have to be limited to that. It's a practice that you can employ throughout various points of the day to induce a state of calm and relief from stress.

PERSONAL STORY

For the longest time, I had a lot of trouble trying to fall asleep. I knew of so many different people who seemingly didn't have any trouble at all when it came to falling asleep. They could simply shut their eyes and fall asleep as if on cue. I noticed that my sleeping problems were greatly affecting my energy levels throughout the day and this wasn't good for my overall productivity. It didn't matter how hard I tried to fall asleep at night. I tried going to bed earlier than I usually did, but I still found my mind rummaging through the most random thoughts well into the night.

I dwelled on the many different circumstances surrounding my life, and I thought about things I should have done differently. I would think about what my future would be like and what I needed to change today in order to achieve all of my dreams. It was like this for me every single day. What ended up happening was that I found myself taking naps at around noon because I always felt so tired in the mornings. I wasn't able to concentrate on work because I knew that I lacked sleep. It felt almost as if I was running on autopilot. Whenever I was communicating with other people, I practically felt like a zombie because I was always so out of it with our conversations.

Ultimately, I decided that enough was enough. I went online and started reading about different theories and solutions surrounding sleep science. I ended up learning a lot, but I was greatly intrigued when I stumbled upon the 4-7-8 method. It seemed simple enough. I mean, how hard is it to breathe, right? It's something that we all do subconsciously every day anyway. There was no harm in trying it in the hopes that it would fix all of my sleep problems. Truth be told, I had much difficulty in the beginning. I wasn't finding as much success as I would have liked. There was something wrong in what I was doing, but I just couldn't put my finger on what it was.

Then, I noticed that there was a slight improvement when I started adopting a more active lifestyle and exercising. I didn't realize that my more active daily routines paired with the breathing exercise dramatically improved my ability to go to sleep earlier at night. After that, I was like a completely different person. I had more energy and wasn't so tired all the time. I had all of the motivation and energy to go and do everything that I set out to do. So, if you're trying this technique out for yourself, don't get discouraged if you don't find immediate success. Sometimes, it takes time before the effects of the exercise can really start to show. Other times, you might have to pair this technique with another habit that is good for promoting your sleep. As we get deeper into this book, we will be discussing other factors that could help improve the quality of your sleep at night.

3

DAILY HABITS

If you find yourself constantly plagued by sleepless nights tossing and turning in your bed, then know that you're not alone. In fact, the National Sleep Foundation determined that around 62% of American adults experience some kind of sleeping issue multiple nights per week. As you may already know, sleep deprivation can snowball into a very serious problem if left unaddressed for too long. Many people innately know just how valuable sleep can be. However, not many people realize that fixing a sleeping problem isn't just a matter of going to bed and forcing yourself to keep your eyes closed.

In this chapter, we are going to talk about all of the habits that make up your daily routine which could potentially be impairing your ability to go to sleep earlier at night. Habits are important because they ultimately determine how your life is going to turn out. Your overall health and success are dependent on the kinds of habits that you employ on a daily basis. This is why it's important for you to familiarize yourself with some of the best and worst habits that you could do for sleep.

WHY HABITS ARE IMPORTANT

According to Charles Duhigg, author of *The Power of Habit*, your habits are very important because they help condition your brain to conduct itself in a certain way. If you are continuously reinforcing bad habits, then you are conditioning your brain to think that this is the right way of doing things even when it's not. For example, you might have a habit of taking in caffeine late in the afternoon. If you do this consistently enough, your brain is going to seek your afternoon coffee even when you know that this isn't going to be good for your quality of sleep.

More importantly, the thing about habits that most people fail to realize is that they are mostly done subconsciously. They are so ingrained into your system and your routine that you don't even realize that you're doing them anymore. It's like brushing your teeth every morning when you wake up and every night before going to sleep. You don't even think about it anymore because it's so deeply ingrained into your routine. It's almost like muscle memory. This is good if the habits you practice are actually helping to improve the quality of your life (such as brushing your teeth). But this can be very problematic if the habits you're practicing are unknowingly compromising the quality of your life.

Again, there may be certain things that you do every day which are making it difficult for you to get a good night's sleep. Since a lot of these things are done habitually, you never really think about them anymore. The example we made earlier about drinking coffee late in the afternoon is rather obvious, and some people might be able to spot that as a problem easily. However, not many people realize that the habit of staring into their phone and computer screens late into the night can impair their ability to get quality sleep as well. You need to be more conscious of how your habits are actually impacting your sleep. This consciousness will lead you to getting rid of any bad habits you might have, and it may also force you to practice good ones in the future.

BAD HABITS THAT ARE COMPROMISING THE QUALITY OF YOUR SLEEP

Okay. So, you're tired of feeling so tired all day, every day. One of the first things that you need to do to correct that problem is to identify all of your bad habits which are contributing to this problem in the first place. Here is a list of some of the most common bad sleeping habits that people typically have.

You're Staring at Screens All Night

It can be very tempting to just mindlessly scroll through your phone, tablet, computer, or TV late at night while you're in bed. After all, your work day is done and it's time for you to relax and unwind, right? What better way to unwind than to engage in mindless media consumption on your preferred devices? Well, it turns out that this seemingly innocent habit is doing much more harm than good. If you've noticed, most modern devices these days come with a blue light filter feature. What this feature does is limit the amount of blue light that a screen is emitting so that it's better for your eyes at night.

But what is blue light and why is it bad for you? Well, blue light in itself is not inherently bad. In fact, the sun, which is the best and most natural source of blue light, is very good for you. It helps wake you up in the morning so that you're more alert and energized to face the day. However, exposure to blue light also has a way of messing up your body's circadian rhythm. Remember earlier when we talked about how your circadian rhythm essentially functions as your own personal body clock? When you're exposing yourself to the blue light that comes from your phone screens at night, it essentially sends signals to your brain telling it that it needs to wake up. This blue light can alter your circadian rhythm by conditioning your body that it's still daytime and it isn't time to go to sleep just yet.

In order to fix this bad habit, try to limit your exposure to blue light in your bedroom. When it comes to lighting fixtures, opt for diffused soft lighting. Aside from that, another obvious fix is to disallow the use of phones and computers in the bedroom at night. If you really want to unwind, grab a book as an alternative to your phone or take on any hobby that doesn't involve you staring at a screen all of the time.

You Drink Too Much Alcohol

You may already be familiar with the concept of a nightcap, wherein people indulge in an alcoholic beverage before bedtime. Some people believe that alcohol helps people fall asleep more easily. While there is some truth to this idea, it's not necessarily the whole story. Ultimately, overindulgence in alcohol prior to bedtime can actually compromise the quality of your sleep.

Yes, there is some truth to the idea that alcohol helps people fall asleep faster. However, what not many people realize is that alcohol can actually keep people from entering into the deep sleep stages of a sleep cycle. We already talked earlier about how it's during the deep sleep stage wherein the body really gets to recover and revitalize itself. If you're unable to stay in a deep sleep for long during the night, you'll still wake up feeling very groggy and tired. This is why it isn't a good idea for you to drink too much alcohol late into the night. Yes, you may fall asleep faster, but you're not getting the kind of sleep that you need to feel energized for the next day.

You Drink Too Much Caffeine

This one should be a rather obvious bad habit that people need to break. We already know that caffeine is a stimulant that is designed to make people feel more alert and awake. This is why it serves as the fuel for people who constantly find themselves feeling too tired or sleepy in the mornings or afternoons at work. Ultimately, coffee in itself isn't bad. In fact, there are many health benefits that are associated with drinking a freshly brewed cup of joe every day. However, there are also certain caveats.

First, you have to consider quantity. Just because it's good for you doesn't mean that you can have however much of it you like. At most, you should only be consuming 400 mg of caffeine per day. That rounds out to about four average-sized cups of coffee. This number can vary from person to person, given that our bodies can respond to caffeine intake in different ways. However, 400 mg should be the hard limit for caffeine intake. If you're drinking any more than that, then you are greatly altering your circadian rhythm to the point where it will be disruptive to your sleep schedule.

Next, you have to consider the timing of your caffeine intake. If you take it too early in the morning, you could potentially end up crashing sometime around noon or a little later. When that happens, you leave yourself susceptible to being groggy and taking a nap. If you take a nap, then this will alter your body's sleep drive. This means that it might be more difficult for you to fall asleep later that night at the time that you're supposed to be sleeping. If you take your caffeine too late in the day, then you risk feeling energized and stimulated well into the night. Even when you're desperate to unwind and relax, the caffeine may still be kicking in and making it difficult for you to fall asleep. This is why you need to make sure that you aren't drinking too much caffeine and that you're taking it during the appropriate parts of the day. Ideally, limit your caffeine intake to less than 400 mg and don't take coffee after 2 p.m.

You Work Out Late in the Night

Exercise and maintaining an active lifestyle is very good for promoting your overall health and wellness. However, as it is with the case of caffeine, just because something is good doesn't mean that you should do it whenever you want. Whenever you engage in any kind of tough exercise, such as lifting weights or going for a run, before you go to bed, it can impact your ability to fall asleep easily. This is because when you engage in vigorous exercise, you are effectively raising the temperature of your body. Also, as you may already know, exercise triggers the release of endorphins, or "happy hormones." Unfortunately, endorphins have a way of making you feel more active and energized. All of these factors combined will make it very hard for you to fall asleep.

Of course, this isn't to say that you shouldn't be exercising. Engaging in an effective and consistent exercise routine is very good for your health, and it can even improve the quality of your sleep. You just want to make sure that you're doing it earlier in the day. At the very least, try to schedule your workouts around two or three hours before your designated bedtime. This will give your body ample time to cool itself down into a more relaxed and sleep-conducive state.

You Eat Too Late at Night

Try to think of how much energy your body needs to generate and exert in order to digest a meal. Your body has to generate this energy within itself in order for your digestive system to function properly. Unfortunately, this metabolic activity will also mean that you might feel a slight boost in your energy directly after a meal. This is why it isn't a good idea for you to eat a big meal particularly close to your bedtime. It's very hard for your body to enter into a relaxed state while it's still digesting food.

Aside from that, lying down while your stomach is digesting can induce a rise of stomach acid into your esophagus. This could lead to uncomfortable sensations brought about by heartburn and indigestion. Have you ever tried falling asleep while battling heartburn and indigestion? It's not easy. Remember that you need to be as comfortable and as relaxed as possible in order for you to fall asleep. Having to deal with discomfort can make this very difficult for you.

GOOD HABITS YOU SHOULD PRACTICE INSTEAD

Getting a good night's sleep isn't just a matter of getting rid of bad habits. You need to take the time to build good habits as well. For this part of the chapter, we are going to talk about some of the best habits that you should incorporate into your daily routines so as to promote better sleep.

Practice a Consistent Sleep Schedule

As much as possible, you want your sleep schedule to be fixed within your daily routine. You want to go to bed and wake up at exactly the same time every single day. This way, your body will gradually condition itself to adjust to the schedule that you set. Not a lot of people realize just how much power and control that they have over their circadian rhythms. You can dramatically alter your body's natural body clock by forcing it to go to sleep and wake up at the same time daily.

Track Your Sleep

One of the best investments you could ever make when you're trying to improve the quality of your sleep is a sleep tracker. Most smartwatches these days are already fitted with some kind of sleep tracking technology, but you can also purchase a dedicated sleep tracker. Ultimately, the goal here is for you to monitor your sleeping habits. Earlier, we talked about how important it is to establish a consistent sleep schedule. Tracking your sleep will allow you further insights into the data surrounding your sleep cycles. This will give you more information into how much sleep you're actually getting and whether you're making the most out of your sleep or not. After all, you might say that you're going to bed at 9:00 p.m., but a sleep tracker will tell you that you're actually falling asleep an hour after that.

Shorten Your Naps

A lot of people demonize naps because they think they'll prevent them from falling asleep later at night. This is true to a certain extent. However, naps can actually be a great way to give yourself a much-needed energy boost in the middle of the day. The key is to make sure that you time your naps properly and that you don't overdo it. Ideally, you would never want to nap for more than 30 minutes every day. Any amount longer than that can compromise the quality of your sleep at night. Aside from that, try to take a nap earlier in the day. If you wake up super early, like 4:00 a.m. or 5:00 a.m., you can take a nap just before noon. Ideally, you wouldn't want to be taking naps too late in the afternoon.

Exercise Early in the Day

Earlier, we talked about how exercising and working out late at night isn't a good idea if you want to fall asleep early. However, you shouldn't take that as an excuse to not exercise at all. We already know that there are many benefits to maintaining an active lifestyle. It helps you lose weight and promotes cardiac health. Aside from that, it lowers stress and anxiety. But you may not know that engaging in a consistent exercise routine can help you sleep easier at night as well.

This is because your body requires a great deal of energy in order to exercise. Naturally, you're using up a lot of your body's calories to perform these movements in rapid succession at an intense pace. It's a given that you're going to feel tired from engaging in such activities. The tiredness and fatigue that you feel from your workouts will actually allow you to fall asleep at night much easier. Just make sure that you're doing it earlier in the day and not right before you sleep.

Establish a Proper Pre-Bedtime Routine

A lot of getting a good night's sleep relies on your brain's activity and mental state. This is why it's good to incorporate conditioning devices into your routine that will try to manipulate your mind into thinking that it's time for bed. It could be any kind of routine at all (as long as it doesn't involve any of the bad habits that we mentioned previously). Following a pre-bedtime routine is a great way of tricking your brain into thinking that it's time to go to bed. Even a simple 30-minute routine can really do wonders. Let's say that you plan to go to bed at 9:00 p.m. Here is a sample 30-minute routine that you could follow:

8:30—Wash face and apply skin care products.

8:40—Perform 10 minutes of light stretching.

8:50—Do a five-minute meditation exercise.

8:55—Turn off the lights in your bedroom and lay down in your bed to prepare to go to sleep at 9:00 p.m.

Of course, your routine doesn't have to look like this. It can even last as long as an hour if you like. Some people like to read in bed in order to tire their eyes out, but this might be counterproductive for others who find themselves staying up late because they want to keep reading. Again, it's all just a matter of finding a routine that works well for you. The most important thing is that you practice it consistently in order for it to be effective.

PERSONAL STORY

There's no denying the fact that the age of social media has drastically affected the way that we do things, both for the good and the bad. In many ways, this age of digital information has made knowledge acquisition and skills development much more accessible. That's definitely a good thing. It's so easy to go online and learn as much as you want about absolutely anything. Learning has never been more accessible or convenient. However, it's not all good when it comes to this new digital age. There are also so many ways that technology hasn't been great for us. One common criticism of mobile technology is that even though it brings us closer to the people who are far from us, it also tends to distance us from those who are immediately around us. It's evident when you're out in public and you see a modern family having dinner together with each of them engrossed in their own devices. Of course, not all people are like this, but it's still a phenomenon that's worth pointing out.

There are a myriad of other ways that technology has negatively affected the way that we live, and one of them is through sleeping. Ever since I got my hands on my first smartphone, I practically went to bed every night with my smartphone in hand. I would just keep on scrolling and scrolling across different social media platforms. Whenever I was done with one, I would hop on over to another site and continue browsing there. Whenever I was done with that, I would hop back to the previous site and keep on scrolling one more time. It was a vicious cycle that I indulged in over and over again without even realizing how much it was affecting my sleep. It didn't feel like I was wasting so much time, but it turns out that I was.

Little did I realize that I was going to sleep as late as midnight or even at 1:30 a.m. I kept this habit for a long time until my body acclimated itself to my schedule. I essentially had a lot of energy until around 1:00 a.m. because my body was used to being up around that time. As you may have guessed, this made it much more challenging for me to wake up early in the mornings. It was always such a struggle for me to drag myself out of bed. More than that, I found myself wanting to have more and more midday naps as well. All of these factors ate away at my productivity. I was groggy and lacked energy, and this made me very inefficient and unfocused with my work. I took a lot of naps, and that took time away from being productive. Most of the time, I felt like I was very demotivated and I didn't have any drive or capacity to develop myself or learn new skills. Aside from that, I found myself making a lot of absent-minded mistakes at work that I didn't typically make. I knew that I was much better than what my performance was showing. I could never pinpoint what the cause of my slump was until I started learning more about the impact of sleep on a person's life. Naturally, I decided to adopt healthier habits, including not using my phone late at night, and I noticed that I was getting many more things done. I was more efficient with my work, and I felt like my life was back on track.

4

"MOVES LIKE JOGGER"

*I*f you have ever been an athlete or if you've tried adopting a structured fitness regimen in the past, you might have had a coach tell you to get enough sleep. We've already talked about the value of sleep when it comes to refreshing, repairing, re-energizing, and revitalizing the human body. This is especially true when the body undergoes any kind of rigorous training program. Yes, sleep is important for athletic performance and fitness. However, the converse is also true. Exercise and being active is also good for the quality of your sleep.

In this chapter, we are going to take a deeper dive into the science of exercise and how it can affect your sleeping habits. Aside from that, we will also dabble into crafting a real exercise routine that you can follow. Don't think you have to be some kind of superpowered athlete in order to reap the benefits of proper exercise. Any kind of structured and intentional movement can be incredibly beneficial for your overall health and wellness, particularly when it comes to sleep. It doesn't matter what age you are or what kind of athletic background you have. You definitely stand to benefit from following a solid exercise routine that you can commit to over an extended period. Aside from that, we'll also talk about some pre-bedtime exercises or stretches that you can incorporate into your nightly routine.

HOW DOES EXERCISE IMPACT SLEEP?

Many researchers and experts have looked into the relationship between sleep and exercise over the years. Of course, this is only a natural curiosity to pursue. After all, we innately know that sleep is when we re-energize ourselves. We also know that exercise requires a lot of energy. It's only natural that these two activities should go hand in hand with one another. Experts believe that not sleeping properly can lead to compromised athletic performance. In addition, studies have also noted that having a proper exercise routine can minimize the effects of sleep-related issues (Pacheco, 2021).

This is why if you're looking to really promote the quality of your sleep, then you need to pay more attention to how you move throughout your day. Sleeping isn't just making sure that you are laying down on a comfortable bed or that your room's AC is set to the right temperature. Again, you also need to consider all of the choices that you make all throughout the day. Truth be told, you shouldn't need much convincing to exercise anyway. Everyone knows that exercise is good for them for a variety of different reasons. It helps develop bone and muscle strength. It aids in improving cardiac and digestive health. It boosts the immune system, and it triggers the release of endorphins (happy hormones). It also helps fight diseases, obesity, and anxiety. On top of all of that, exercise also helps you sleep better.

To be more specific, you should look to incorporate moderate to vigorous exercise into your daily routine as much as you can. It's been shown that exercise can dramatically increase the quality of your sleep while also allowing you to fall asleep quicker and earlier in the night. This means that you won't waste as much time tossing and turning in bed at night. Also, since exercise triggers the release of endorphins, it can also leave you feeling more energized throughout the day. This will decrease the likelihood of you wanting to nap.

Exercise has another more subtle and indirect way of improving one's quality of sleep. We all know that one of the major benefits of having an active lifestyle is that it helps us stay trim and lean. We also probably know that there are many serious physical health conditions that are associated with weight gain and obesity. But what not a lot of people realize is that having excess fat in the body can also increase the likelihood of experiencing the symptoms of obstructive sleep apnea (OSA). This is a condition that makes it challenging for people to gather oxygen while in a sleeping state. The lack of oxygen can result in a person's inability to get into the deep sleep stage of a cycle where processes of recuperation and recovery take place. Around 60% of cases of moderate to severe OSA are known to be attributed to obesity (Pacheco, 2021).

Interestingly enough, the National Sleep Foundation conducted a poll back in 2003 that involved adults between the ages of 55 and 84. The survey found that around 52% of respondents admitted to exercising three or more times per week while 24% said that they exercised less than once a week. The study also found that those who fell under the latter category were more likely to not get even six hours of sleep per night. That's two hours less than the recommended eight hours of sleep. Aside from that, these people were also more likely to experience sleeping problems such as insomnia, sleep apnea, and restlessness at night.

In a more recent poll by Sleep in America that was conducted in 2013, adults between the ages of 23 and 60 were surveyed. Unsurprisingly, the survey yielded somewhat similar results to the 2003 study that was conducted by the NSF. This survey found that 76-83% of respondents who engaged in either light, moderate, or vigorous exercise routines admitted to having either very good or fairly good sleep quality. However, for those who didn't exercise as often or as regularly, only around 56% of respondents said the same. Regardless of the age, it was found that people who exercised more regularly were also more likely to get more and better quality sleep than others. Others who are less active are more likely to have irregular sleep and in other words be a couch potato.

EXERCISING FOR BETTER SLEEP

Now, we are going to try to develop a proper exercise plan that you can stick to in order to improve the quality of your sleep and just the quality of your life in general as well. However, before we get into the details, it's important to preface this section of the book by saying that you should always consult a doctor or a licensed trainer before embarking on any kind of exercise routine. This is especially true if you have limited experience when it comes to exercise and fitness in general. Given that, all of the information that will be listed in this book is still based on sound research and best practices.

Aerobic vs Anaerobic Exercise

Before you can think about crafting an exercise routine for yourself, there's something that you need to learn: the difference between aerobic and anaerobic exercise. Even if you're not particularly interested in fitness, you might already be familiar with these two terms. But what exactly do they mean?

Aerobic exercise is any kind of intentional and structured physical activity that is designed to strengthen your cardiac health. Often, aerobic exercises are what people in the fitness community refer to as 'cardio.' In any kind of aerobic workout, you are engaging in an activity that slightly elevates your heart rate, making it somewhat difficult for you to carry a conversation. This is because your body is hard at work trying to process as much oxygen as it can to sustain your movements. But the rate of your movements during aerobic exercise are controlled so that you are able to sustain them for much longer. Some common examples of aerobic exercise include running, brisk walking, jumping jacks, jumping rope, cycling, and rowing.

Anaerobic exercise consists of movements designed to really get your heart pumping at a massive pace. It's practically impossible to carry a conversation with someone when you're operating within the anaerobic threshold. It's also unlikely that you would be able to sustain any kind of anaerobic movement for too long. This causes a buildup of lactic acid in your blood which will make it difficult for your muscles to be oxygenated. Some examples of anaerobic exercise include burpees, Olympic lifts, squats, kettlebell swings, and sprinting. These are rapid movements that often require a great deal of intensity and are typically performed in bursts.

When it comes to fat loss, it's typically believed that anaerobic workouts are more efficient for promoting fat burn. In all practicality, both aerobic and anaerobic exercises are designed to promote caloric burn. The more calories you burn, the more fat you burn in the process. However, the key difference lies in *how* these two fitness paradigms approach calorie-burning. When it comes to aerobic exercise, you're only ever really burning calories as long as you're sustaining the movement. You elevate your heart rate and recruit your various muscle groups to put your body into motion. All of these things dramatically increase the amount of calories that you need to burn within that time. However, once you stop and your body's heart rate returns to normal, you burn the same amount of calories as you typically would.

On the other hand, with anaerobic exercise, you're typically engaging in a process that dramatically strains your muscles to the point of breakage. For example, when you're lifting heavy weights, you break a lot of your muscle fibers that need to be filled in with protein. Once these breakages are filled in, the muscle comes back bigger and stronger. This is the science of bodybuilding. It's a constant process of breaking to build. The reason this is also much more effective for fat loss is that it allows for your body to burn more calories even when your body is at rest. Unlike with aerobic exercises, once you're done with your aerobic workout, your body is still working hard to repair itself and recover from the exercise. This means that it's using up more calories over the entire course of a day or two (depending on how intense the workout is). So, your body ends up burning more calories over time even when you're no longer working out.

But when it comes to sleep, what's better? Should you opt for aerobic or anaerobic exercise? According to a recent study, both aerobic and anaerobic exercise can greatly improve the quality of one's sleep (Saber et al., 2017). However, the same study also found that people who engaged in consistent anaerobic exercise were found to have a greater quality of sleep than those who merely engaged in aerobic training. Despite this, it's important to note that the disparity between these two groups was not all that significant. The real takeaway from the study was that any kind of exercise did much for improving sleep quality, regardless of whether it was aerobic or anaerobic.

How Much Exercise Is Enough?

The answer to this question is tricky depending on the kind of lifestyle you have. When it comes to fitness training, the needs of any person vary only by degrees, but not by kind. Everyone needs to exercise, but everyone will have varying levels of requirements when it comes to the training they engage in. For example, a professional athlete will need to spend more hours at the gym compared to a 60-year-old retiree who is just looking to stay active. Both of these people need to maintain a proper fitness regimen, but one will have a significantly higher workload than the other.

Typically, it's recommended that one engages in around 30 to 60 minutes of exercise for three to five days per week. As much as possible, you want to balance your exercise regimen out by incorporating healthy doses of both aerobic and anaerobic training. Aerobic training is better for promoting cardiac health, respiratory health, endurance, and stamina. Anaerobic training is better for promoting fat loss, strength, agility, and explosiveness. Both of these exercise paradigms have their individual strengths, and they both aid in improving the quality of your sleep as well. Also, mixing up your training regimen will make your healthy habits more sustainable. People tend to stick to their healthy lifestyles more when they are not repetitive or predictable. That being said, developing a workout schedule is vital for a healthy body.

A Reminder About Exercising Before Bed

There have been many discussions among experts over the years regarding how many hours prior to bed one should engage in exercise. Most experts in the field of sleep science believe that engaging in vigorous exercise within a three-hour period prior to sleep can negatively affect one's quality of rest. This is because exercise can increase a person's heart rate while raising their body temperature and adrenaline levels. All of these factors contribute to a compromised quality of sleep. However, there are also experts in the field whose studies have led them to believe that exercising prior to sleep doesn't produce as negative an effect as most people might think.

One study found that people who exercise around 8 p.m. or later tend to fall asleep quicker. They are also documented to have gotten an adequate amount of deep sleep, which is a stage of sleep that is crucial for energy recuperation and recovery (Youngstedt & Kline, 2006). This study was done with a group that was contrasted against another group that worked out between the hours of 4 and 8 p.m. The group that worked out during earlier hours were found to report similar effects as those who worked out at later times.

However, in one survey that was commissioned by the National Sleep Foundation back in 2005, it was found that adults aged 18 and older were highly unlikely to work out during the later parts of the day. Only around 4% of respondents said that they exercised within an hour of going to sleep every night.

This is the reason why those in the sleep science and hygiene community continue to be so divided on the matter. In principle, working out later at night has all of the ingredients to compromise one's sleep. And yet, there are persistent studies that show that working out later at night doesn't have that significant of an impact on a person's sleep. Regardless, if you're a person who would rather err on the side of safety, it would be better to plot your workouts during the earlier parts of the day. This will give your body ample time to relax before it's actually time for you to go to bed.

Pre-Bedtime Stretches and Exercises

With everything that has been said so far, not all forms of exercise are typically bad. In fact, many people like to incorporate mild stretches and movements into their pre-bedtime routine. While the idea of engaging in intense workouts directly before bedtime is still hotly contested, there's really no harm in doing a few stretches to help you relax before sleeping. In fact, aside from getting your regular dose of exercise, stretching just before bed can help you relax and calm your mind.

Stretching is a great alternative to you just scrolling through social media while you're in bed. This will disrupt your sleep and circadian rhythm because of the dopamine releases and the blue light emissions from your computer or phone screen. It would be much better to have your pre-bedtime routine be composed of stretches that are designed to lengthen and relax your muscles so that they are better primed for sleeping.

Aside from that, stretching has a way of promoting the positive effects of meditation on your body. It will allow you to center your focus on both your breathing and your muscle's sensations. This will take your mind away from everything that might be stressing you out or causing you any anxieties. This level of mindfulness is proven to be able to relax you and help induce a state of calmness which can aid in getting you to fall asleep quicker. This is all in addition to the practical and physical benefits of stretching, such as relieving muscle tension and tightness.

Here are a few stretches and exercises that you may want to consider incorporating into your routine.

Knee to Chest

The knee to chest stretch is a great pose to perform while you're already lying down in bed. It's designed to alleviate any pressure that might be present within your hip joint, especially with your hip flexor. It's also a great way of decompressing your lower back, where a lot of tension tends to get built up during the day. With this stretch, you will focus on just one knee at a time.

1. Lie done with your back completely flat and your head facing towards the ceiling.
2. Gently lift one leg and bend it at the knee.

3. Clasp both your hands around the front of your knee cap and pull your knee towards your chest.
4. Try to get deeper into the stretch with every exhale. Remember to be mindful of your breathing throughout the entire process.
5. Hold the pose for the duration of 30 seconds or five full breaths.
6. Release the pose and repeat the process on the other leg. Perform around three to five sets on each leg.

Spinal Twist

The spinal twist is another great pose that you can perform while you're already lying down on your bed. This is very effective at helping release any knots that may exist within your lower back. Expect to hear a few cracks from your lower back when you get into this stretch. That's completely normal and is a part of the decompression process. Aside from that, this is a great pose for promoting range of motion within the hip joint while also stretching out the IT band.

1. Start by laying yourself down so that you are facing towards the ceiling.
2. Like in the previous stretch, gently lift one leg and bend it at the knee.
3. Using your opposite hand, grab the outer side of your lifted leg and gently pull it towards the opposite side. Try to make your femur perpendicular to your body.
4. Be mindful of your breathing throughout the entire stretch and try to get deeper into the pose with every exhale.
5. It's also important that you don't rotate your torso as

this will undo the rotation that should be taking place within the hip joint.
6. Hold the stretch for around 30 seconds and repeat for a total of three to five sets.

Child's Pose

Child's pose is a popular yoga stretch that is also commonly known as the prayer pose. It's designed to induce a sense of relaxation and decompression within the body. Typically, instructors will suggest to beginner yogis to get into a child's pose whenever they feel like they can't keep up with the natural flow or movement of the class. It requires very little effort to get into, and it's great for promoting relaxation and blood flow within the body while also reducing stress and tension in the back, shoulders, and neck.

1. Start the pose by getting into a kneeling position on the floor. Feel free to place pads or a yoga mat underneath your knees for added support.
2. Sit back on your heels and maintain a fully neutral upright position.
3. Spread your knees outward and hinge at your hips as you tilt yourself forward.
4. Try to fold forward as far as you can by reaching your arms outwards in front of you. Grab a hold of the ground with your palms and try to pull yourself deeper into the stretch. Aim to get your forehead as close to the floor as possible.
5. Be mindful of your breathing throughout the entire pose and try to get deeper into the stretch with every exhale.

6. Hold the pose for around 30 seconds or five full breaths before repeating for a total of three to five sets.

Sphinx Pose

The sphinx pose is another great way to relieve a lot of the pressure that gets built up within the mid and lower back. It creates an exaggerated arch in the spine so as to counteract any hunching of the back that people tend to hold for prolonged periods throughout the course of the day. The stretch also provides the added benefit of strengthening and stabilizing the shoulder joint.

1. Start the stretch by lying down on your stomach with your legs extended straight out behind you.
2. Place your elbows directly underneath your shoulders with your forearms flat on the floor and your fingers pointed forward.
3. Using your forearms as stabilizers, push yourself up so that your chest is lifted off the floor.
4. As your chest gets lifted up, you should feel a slight stretch in your mid and lower back.
5. Be mindful of your breathing throughout the entire pose and try to elongate your spine further with every exhale.
6. Be careful not to overextend your back to the point wherein you feel any kind of pain. Remember that slight discomfort is normal when you're stretching, but you should never be in pain.

Butterfly Pose

The butterfly pose is a great way to open up your hips just before you go to sleep at night. It is also a relatively easy pose to get into, and it requires very minimal effort on your part to really feel the effects of the stretch. Aside from opening up your hips, the butterfly pose also helps relieve some of the tension within the lower back that can arise as a result of poor sitting positions.

1. Start the pose by sitting on the floor with your legs extended straight out in front of you.
2. Make sure that your butt is planted firmly on the floor as you bend both of your knees and bring the two soles of your feet together.
3. Use your hands to bring both your feet into your body towards your groin area.
4. Gently hinge at your hips and lean forward to get deeper into the stretch. Make sure to maintain a neutral spine throughout the entire process and be mindful of not hunching your back.
5. Be mindful of your breathing throughout the entire pose and try to get deeper into the stretch with every exhale.
6. Hold the pose for around 30 seconds or five full breaths and repeat for a total of three to five sets.

Bear Hug

The bear hug stretch is designed to work on the rhomboids and the trap muscles of your upper back. This is a great way to promote the range of motion of your shoulder joint while also relieving your scapula of any discomfort or tightness. A lot of the time, a person's shoulder joint can get compromised by poor posture while working on a desk the whole day. The bear hug is a great way to counteract all of that stress within the shoulder joint while relieving pressure within that entire region of the body.

1. Stand in a fully upright position with a neutral spine and your feet directly underneath your hips.
2. Exhale deeply as you cross your arms and reach your hands to your back as if you were giving yourself a hug.
3. Be mindful of your breathing and allow yourself to get deeper into the stretch with every exhale.
4. Hold the stretch for around 30 seconds or five full breaths.
5. Release the pose on your final exhale and repeat for another three to five sets.

PERSONAL STORY

When the COVID-19 pandemic first broke out back in the earlier parts of the year 2020, people started paying much more attention to their health and wellness. Understandably, this is a natural response that any rational being might have to the emergence of a global pandemic and health emergency. For my part, I decided to try running laps around three times a week to strengthen my lungs and my cardiovascular system. In my mind, this was the best way for me to protect myself against the disease. After all, COVID-19 at that time was understood to wreak havoc on a person's respiratory system. So, I figured if I strengthened my lungs as much as possible, I would give myself a fighting chance against the disease.

However, what I didn't anticipate was that exercising consistently also managed to improve the other aspects of my life. Yes, I felt a lot stronger, and I had more energy as a result of my improved fitness. I also found that a lot of the sleeping problems that I was experiencing were being addressed as well. I always found myself so tired at the end of the day as a result of my increased physical activity. Running required so much energy from my body that I found myself just crashing on my bed every night without even trying. It was so much easier for me to fall asleep. It was also so natural and so sudden. I went from being someone who had to consciously force myself to go to sleep every night with little success to someone who was practically out like a light in just a matter of a couple of minutes.

5

WHEN IN ROOM

hen in room… do as the roomans do? Okay, that doesn't make any sense. What I'm trying to say here is that if you really want to enhance the quality of your sleep, you can't just look inward at what you're doing. Your immediate environment also has a lot to do with how fast you drift off into dreamland and how long you can stay asleep as well. In most cases, your immediate sleeping environment should be your bedroom. This is why this chapter is going to take a more focused look into how you should set up your bedroom so that it's primed to become an optimal sleeping environment.

Take note that there are some people who can seemingly fall asleep at will regardless of where they are. However, some kinds of people are very particular about the sleeping environment that they're in. This is the reason why some people struggle with going to sleep whenever they find themselves in hotels or any kind of unfamiliar territory. These minute changes in the environment can really do a lot in altering a person's sleep psychology. You may not have paid attention to these things before, but various factors like lighting and air temperature do impact your overall sleep health.

It's very important that you structure your environment in a way that promotes a good night's sleep. It doesn't matter what kind of habits you employ during the day. Even if you cut back on your caffeine intake or refrain from taking naps, if your room is not optimized for sleeping, then you're still going to experience a few issues here and there.

Before we delve into the details, it's also important that you realize that you don't necessarily have to spend your entire life's savings on remodeling your room so that it becomes optimized for sleeping. There are just a few minor tweaks or changes that you need to make in order to make sure that your bedroom becomes a conducive environment for promoting a good night's sleep.

TEMPERATURE

Whether it's obvious to you or not, the temperature of your sleeping environment can have a significant impact on both the length and quality of your sleep. This is because your body's temperature goes down whenever it falls asleep. Essentially, your brain is programmed so that it thinks that your body is supposed to start falling asleep when it reaches a certain temperature. So, creating the ideal temperature within your sleeping environment will send signals to your brain telling it that it's time to start shutting down so that you can transition into a sleeping state.

Conversely, if your body is within an environment that is either too warm or too cool, then it will make it difficult for your brain to distinguish whether it's time for you to start falling asleep or not. However, given the fact that your body's temperature lowers when you sleep, it's much easier to fall asleep in an environment that is cooler rather than warmer. Aside from helping you fall asleep quicker, having the ideal temperature in a room will allow your body to stay asleep longer so that you get the full benefits of each stage of the sleeping cycle.

Ultimately, there is no magic number for everyone when it comes to the ideal temperature for sleeping environments. We all have different bodies that have different temperatures at any given time. This is where the art of trial and error comes in. Most experts will say that it's best to keep your room at a temperature somewhere between 65 and 72 degrees Fahrenheit. However, the ultimate truth is that you just need to find the optimal temperature that works best for your body. Again, all of our bodies respond in a variety of different ways.

When it comes to temperature, there are many tools or variables that you need to take into consideration. For the most part, when it comes to regulating room temperature, people might only consider radiators or air conditioning units. However, there are other factors that come into play, such as the materials of your bed sheets or your blankets. Even your sleeping apparel can play a big role in determining the temperature of your body.

LIGHTING

Your human body functions more like a machine than you would think. Over the years, human beings have evolved to synchronize their natural body clocks or circadian rhythms with the rotation of the earth. Whenever the sun rises, your biological clock is primed for energy and activity, and whenever it sets, your body starts winding down for the day. This is why it's especially important that you pay closer attention to the way that you light your home, particularly your bedroom.

We've already talked earlier about how your exposure to light can greatly impact the way that your body's circadian rhythm is formatted. In particular, there are three specific aspects of light exposure that you want to pay attention to: color, brightness, and timing. If you are able to master these factors effectively, then you will be able to prime your body in such a way that it's only exposed to the type of light that's conducive for a specific time of the day.

Before we can talk about the specifics, let's do a deep review of how light can impact the way that your circadian rhythm functions. Again, during the day, the sun gives off a very bright blue-light emission. Once your eye absorbs this light and processes it in your mind, it perceives this light as a signal for you to be more alert and awake. It makes you feel more energized because of melatonin suppression. Melatonin is a hormone in your brain that gets released over time and is responsible for making you feel sleepy. However, the more exposure you have to blue light, the more your brain will suppress the release of melatonin so that you can stay awake for longer. This is why it's particularly effective to expose yourself to natural sunlight early in the morning right when you wake up. This will help reset your brain so that it becomes more primed to start the day.

At night, your brain doesn't get much exposure to natural sunlight anymore and the melatonin levels in your body will gradually rise. They will eventually get to a point wherein you feel so sleepy that it becomes increasingly difficult for you to keep your eyes open. However, if there is a lot of artificial light in your home or in your bedroom that mimics the blue light that comes from the sun, then this will impede the release of melatonin in your body and make it harder for you to enter that sleepy state.

LED bulbs are great for use during the day because they are so good at replicating the bright natural light from the sun. Aside from that, they are incredibly energy efficient. However, once night rolls around, you want to limit your exposure to blue light as much as possible. So, avoid any rooms in your home that may expose you to blue light emissions. You also want to avoid the screens on your phones, tablets, or computers because they are typically programmed to emit blue light as well.

These days, there are so many companies that produce color-changing smart LED bulbs that you can program for various points throughout the day. As much as possible, keep the lights warm and dim at night. This means that you should opt for color hues that fall within the red or orange spectrum. Try to mimic the natural glow of candlelight within your home.

NOISE

This may already be obvious to you, but noise also plays a big role in the quality of your sleep. When you are exposed to too much noise, it can have the same kinds of effects as prolonged exposure to blue light. Think of the last time that you tried to fall asleep during a noisy commotion. Maybe your next-door neighbor was throwing a party. Maybe a family member in another part of the house was watching a movie with the volume at full blast. Whatever the case, it probably wasn't easy for you, right?

Well, as it turns out, having a quiet environment devoid of noise isn't just important to helping you fall asleep. It's also crucial to ensuring that you reap the full benefits of each stage of the sleep cycle. When you try to sleep and there's constant noise in the background, it can actually prevent you from getting into the deeper stages of the sleep cycle. This means that you won't get to experience the rejuvenative processes of the deep sleep stage as much if noise is constantly disrupting your sleep.

Also, it's important to note that the noise that we're talking about here is the kind that is disruptive and hard to ignore. There are other kinds of noise, such as white noise, which some experts say can even help induce sleepiness. White noise acts as if it's playing in the background of your life, and you typically don't even notice it. Examples of white noise include the humming of your air-conditioning unit or the splatter of the rain. You can hear these things when you try to listen to them. But if you don't pay them any attention, then you forget that they're even there. The goal of getting to sleep properly is to block out every other kind of noise such as the ones we mentioned earlier.

Here are a few things that you can do for your bedroom to isolate your room from disruptive noises.

- Add lots of soft surfaces to your room, like curtains and sheets. Fabrics tend to do very well at absorbing any surrounding sound. This means that they help weaken sound waves so that by the time these waves get to your ears, they are completely faint or gone altogether.
- Put all of your electronic devices to silent mode. Some phones have a vibrate mode, and it's important to note that vibrating sounds can be just as disruptive

as ringtones. So, make it a rule to put your phone on silent mode at night so that you aren't disrupted by vibrations or sounds while you sleep.

- Wear ear plugs. If you really can't avoid being surrounded by noise (maybe you live in an area that throws a lot of parties at night), then you might want to invest in a proper set of ear plugs. This will do a great job at blocking out any external sound. This might take some getting used to as the ear plugs will feel awkward at first, but you will eventually warm up to them over time.

BEDDING, PILLOWS, AND MATTRESS

To conclude this chapter, we will be discussing the various parts of your environment that have direct physical contact with your body: your bedding, pillows, and mattress. If you're young and don't really experience too many aches and pains yet, then picking out the right mattress and pillows might not matter much to you. However, if you have back and neck problems all the time, you probably know just how much a good mattress and pillow set can make a difference. This doesn't just have to do with the physiology of your body. It also has a lot to do with the quality of your sleep. We've already gone through so much trouble in making sure that the lighting, temperature, and sound environment of our room is optimal for sleeping. Why wouldn't you devote as much care and attention to the items that are in direct contact with your skin? Of course, each person's bed is always going to be different. Some people prefer adjustable beds while others have warmers or coolers set into their mattresses. Sleep technology development is at an all-time high, and there are so many new tools and devices coming out that are designed to promote sleep. But for now, we're going to focus on the basics that people typically tend to have the most access to.

Mattress

Let's start with the mattress. When you're shopping for a mattress for the first time, you might not be prepared for how comprehensive the options can get. Commercial mattresses are literally sold in all sorts of different shapes and sizes. They are also made out of different materials. Some mattresses are made out of the popular memory foam material while others are made out of hard springs. Given all of these options, it might be hard to actually come to a decision on what specific mattress to buy and which one would be best for your personal sleeping style.

The first thing you need to consider about a mattress is its size. Will you be sleeping alone? Will you be sharing the bed with someone else? Typically, if you're someone who wants to save space in your room, you might want to get a mattress that's small and perfect just for you. However, if you will be sharing the bed with someone else, it would be best to splurge on a bigger mattress as sleep real estate is very important when it comes to the quality of sleep. You don't want to be in the middle of drifting into a deep sleep only to have it interrupted by your partner accidentally whacking you across the face because of the lack of space.

The next detail you want to consider is the material of the mattress. When it comes to choosing material, there are two additional considerations you want to make: comfort and durability. Some materials are designed to be as soft as possible while others are designed to be more structured and supportive. Some materials also need to be replaced more often than others. There is no one particular mattress material that is the definitive best as it all depends on a variety of factors like your sleep position, personal preference, and budget as well. Let's run through all of the most popular mattress materials and who they are best for.

1. Foam. Foam mattresses, particularly those made out of memory foam, tend to be the more popular options for mattress materials these days. This is because memory foam tends to offer a lot of comfort while also being durable enough to last many years. These foam mattresses are designed to adjust and counter themselves to the shape of the body. This is why it's a great option for people who tend to be lighter and who sleep on their sides, where their weight isn't thoroughly distributed all throughout the body.

2. Innerspring. Innerspring or spring mattresses are also very popular, especially among the heavier sleepers. They offer more support than other mattress materials and tend to be the preferred option for people who like to sleep on their backs or stomachs. Spring mattresses are bouncier, and they are also typically cheaper than foam mattresses as well. That's what makes them more appealing to budget-conscious shoppers.

3. Latex. Out of all the mattress materials, latex is the most durable option. These mattresses are made out of a latex rubber material (hence its name) and are bouncier and more durable than innerspring mattresses. Not a lot of people are a fan of the softer latex material as opposed to foam, so it's not particularly popular among the masses. However, it is a great choice for those who are looking for a little

extra support at night while they sleep without completely compromising comfort.

4. Hybrid. Lastly, we have hybrid mattresses. Consider this as the 'Goldilocks' of mattress materials. It's the best of both worlds for people who like the comfort and softness of foam while also craving the support and firmness of innerspring materials. The innersprings are typically located at the bottom parts of the mattress while the foam parts are located at the top so that they are able to contour to the sleeper's body.

Now, when it comes to choosing the right mattress for you, this is the general rule of thumb: the lighter you are, the softer the mattress material should be. This is why kids' mattresses tend to be made out of soft foam or even feathers. As you age and get heavier, your body will require a little more support while you sleep. Also, if you tend to sleep on your side, that means that there's less surface contact between your body and the mattress. Opt for softer mattresses if you are a side sleeper. However, with more surface contact from sleeping on your back or front, then you need something with a little more support, like a foam or a hybrid solution.

All in all, the best way to find the perfect mattress for you is to go to the mattress store and try one out for yourself. Get a good feel for the mattress and pay close attention to how your body responds to it. Remember that you will be sleeping on top of this thing for years. This shouldn't be a decision that you rush or take lightly. Your future self will thank you for whatever time and effort you put into making your buying decision.

Pillows

The next item that we should be discussing is pillows. As with mattresses, your pillows can also be made up of different shapes, sizes, and materials. Again, there is no one definitive pillow for everyone as we all sleep differently. In this part of the chapter, we will be talking about the various pillow options that are available to you and which one would suit your personal sleeping style the best.

Before we can get to discussing your options, remind yourself of what a pillow's job is really supposed to be. Ultimately, a pillow functions as a support system for your preferred sleeping position. Just because a pillow feels soft or comfortable doesn't necessarily mean that it's going to support the way that you sleep. At the end of the day, a pillow should complement the way that your head, neck, and spine are positioned while you sleep. When it comes to choosing materials like this, the rule of thumb is to choose the one that you notice the least while you sleep. If you don't notice it while you're lying down, that means that it's doing its job effectively. If you do notice it while you're using it, then that means that something is off with the way that the device (whether pillow or mattress) is serving your body.

Again, like we discussed in the previous section about mattresses, the pillows you choose should be in service to your preferred sleeping position. Aside from that, your choice of pillows should also depend on whether you tend to run warm or cool while you sleep. Some pillows are made out of materials that tend to expel or keep heat more efficiently. You also have to consider the budget as these pillows can get really pricey sometimes.

For Back Sleepers

If you're a back sleeper, then you want a pillow that sits right within the middle of the spectrum when it comes to comfort and height. You don't want a pillow that's too tall as this can impact the curvature of your neck and leave you fatigued after a night of sleeping. You also don't want a pillow that's too soft to support your head appropriately to maintain that neutral spine. When choosing a pillow, opt for one with a *medium loft* and *medium firmness*.

For Side Sleepers

If you're a side sleeper, then you should look to getting a pillow that offers more in terms of loft and firmness. You want a taller pillow because this is going to help prop your head up to a point where it maintains a neutral alignment with your spine. Aside from that, having a taller pillow will help take some of the pressure off your shoulders while you sleep. This can lessen the likelihood of you developing any tightness or soreness within your neck and shoulder areas.

When it comes to firmness, you want a pillow that offers substantial support so as to make sure that your neck doesn't sink too deeply into the cushion at night. This will prevent your neck from tilting more towards one particular side and will allow you to be more comfortable while you sleep. Having the wrong pillow is one of the major reasons that people develop a stiff neck in the morning.

For Stomach Sleepers

Lastly, if you sleep on your stomach, you should find a pillow with a low profile and that is as soft as possible. While you sleep on your stomach, you are placing your neck in a somewhat awkward position that it isn't used to being in. You can alleviate that awkwardness by making use of a pillow with a lower loft so that you aren't craning your head too much to the point that you're straining it. Again, the whole point of the pillow is that it should naturally complement your preferred sleeping position.

Aside from the pillow being low in profile, it should also be softer. When you sleep on your stomach, you don't want a pillow with too much support, especially when it is in direct contact with your face. You want a pillow that offers a sinking sensation, especially when you are pressing your face against it. Aside from that, a softer profile will also ensure the proper alignment of your neck and spine.

Shapes and Sizes

There are also specialty pillows that can be used for other parts of your body. For example, some people need a little more support in their lower back. There are specially designed pillows that offer lumbar support while you sleep. There are also people, particularly side sleepers, who need pillows at their sides to rest their arms upon. Back sleepers might need specialized pillows to support their legs. Again, your best option would be to hop on over to a nearby store and try the pillows on for size. You might find that a lot of these pillows are more expensive than you initially thought, but they can sometimes be worth the investment. Like mattresses, you will be using these items literally every single day over the next few years. You might as well splurge on something of high quality that you won't have to replace every so often. Aside from that, the pricier pillows also tend to be the ones that literally help you sleep better at night.

Bedding

We've already talked about how the right mattress can help provide support or comfort to your body while you sleep. Choosing the wrong mattress will increase the likelihood of a number of issues, including lower back pain. A pillow is also crucial for your sleep quality as they are supposed to ensure the proper alignment of your neck and spine. However, there is one more crucial detail that you need to consider when you're shopping for your bed, and that's your bedding. A lot of people just choose their beddings nonchalantly. They go for whatever looks good or whatever matches the aesthetics of their room. Not to say that visual design doesn't matter, but there are also other more functional aspects of a bedding material that you need to take into consideration.

Material

If your body temperature tends to be on the cooler side and you require more warmth while you sleep, then you can opt for microfiber bedsheets. They do a good job at retaining heat while still being relatively breathable. They also tend to be very inexpensive while being easy to maintain as well. This makes them a great option for those who are operating within a budget.

On the other hand, if your body temperature tends to run a little warm, then you want a material that is as cool and breathable as possible. If that's the case, then you should go for pure cotton bed sheets. Now, it's important to note that not all cotton is created equal. Typically, the higher-end cottons are Pima cotton and Egyptian cotton. Although these two variations also tend to come with a heftier price tag, they offer the most comfort and coolness, especially for those who live in warmer climates. There is also sateen-finished cotton, which isn't as cool but is incredibly soft to the touch. One major problem with natural cotton is that it absorbs a lot of moisture. So, it wouldn't be a good option for people who are particularly sweaty. Fortunately, there are some moisture-wicking cotton fabrics out there that would be a great alternative.

Thread Count

Aside from the material of the bedding, another factor you might want to pay attention to is the thread count. On the lower end of the spectrum, typical bed sheets will have a thread count of around 300 to 400. That isn't necessarily bad, and it tends to get the job done for most people. There is also a false assumption that the higher a bedding's thread count, the better the sleeping experience is going to be. However, that isn't necessarily the case. A lot of the time, beddings with higher thread counts will compensate by making use of lower-quality fabrics. In this instance, it would be better to go for the bedding with a lower thread count that's made of a high-quality material. Ultimately, the material of a fabric is a much more important factor than its thread count.

Seasonal Bedding

If you live in a seasonal area, then you might want to invest in different fabrics for your beddings. During the warmer months of the year, opt for cottons that are breathable and will allow you to stay cool while you sleep. During the colder parts of the year, go for heavier fabrics like microfiber that will help retain more heat so that you won't wake up shivering in the middle of the night.

PERSONAL STORY

This chapter may have been a lot to take in, especially when you're new to the whole concept of sleep science. That's fine. It's okay to feel overwhelmed. In my own personal experience, it really took me a lot of trial and error to figure out how to optimize my sleep experience based on my own personal preferences. I took my time to really dial in on what my body responded best to, and that wasn't a quick process at all. There were so many factors that I needed to take into consideration, but I found that all of the effort became worth it over time.

In terms of temperature, I've had the benefit (or curse) of experiencing both extremes. During the days of my youth, I did not grow up in a particularly wealthy household. As much as possible, we made conscious efforts to keep the electricity bills down. Naturally, this included limiting the use of heaters and air conditioners in our home. During the winter months, I typically wanted the home to be warmed up to around 75 to 77 degrees Fahrenheit. However, in an effort to cut costs, my family typically kept the heater at around 68 degrees. At first glance, this might not seem like it makes that much of a difference. I decided to compensate for the colder temperatures by bundling up in layers of clothes and blankets. Even when I did that, I still found myself going to bed feeling really cold. It was a struggle for me to go to sleep when my feet were practically shivering. As I got older and started earning my own money, I decided to use some of that cash to solve the problem. One of the first things that I bought was a heating blanket that I lay down on. This definitely helped keep me warm during the winter months. Then, I also had a fuzzy blanket that I used to cover up. The blanket was placed in between my body and a normal comforter that insulated everything. To top it all off, I wore special thick socks to bed to help keep my feet warm. If it got particularly cold, I would sometimes even wear a warm fuzzy robe to bed for some added layers. I can definitely say that investing more of my time and money into these special tools and devices have dramatically improved the quality of my sleep. Not only did I start falling asleep a lot quicker, but I also ended up staying asleep far longer.

When it came to the mattress that I was using, it took me a few years to figure out what my body wanted the most. Eventually, I found that I mostly preferred a mattress that was on the firmer side. Again, my family wasn't particularly well off when I was growing up. This meant that my parents couldn't really afford to buy me new mattresses. I believe the mattress that I slept on while I was growing up was probably around 20 years old at that point. I've tried sleeping on mattresses with springs that didn't offer as much bounce and support as they should have. I've also tried sleeping on mattresses that were so soft that I felt like I was sinking deeper and deeper into quicksand every night I went to bed. Once I had enough money to actually afford a mattress of my own, I visited my nearby IKEA and tried out every single mattress that they had. Eventually, I discovered that for my sleeping style, I preferred a firmer feel to the mattresses, and that's what I've gone with ever since.

6

CONSUMING BEHAVIOR

Who would have known that the food you eat could also impact the way that you sleep? When people go on diets, they typically do so because they either want to lose weight or build their muscles. Some people go on diets to improve their cardiac health or blood sugar levels. However, it's very rare to encounter a person who sticks to a strict diet because it helps them sleep better at night.

As you may have already ascertained throughout the course of reading this book so far, there are so many factors to consider when it comes to shaping the quality of your sleeping experience. We've already talked about how factors like environment and exercise are important in determining the quality of your sleep. You might as well add diet to that list too.

Earlier, we touched on how it's a bad idea for you to consume any caffeine too late in the day. Naturally, caffeine is a stimulant that will make you feel more awake and more alert. This is why you want to avoid taking it so close to your bedtime. Not too many people are aware that eating a greasy burger or a plate of fries before bedtime might not be such a good idea either. In this chapter, we are going to go over the nuances of how your diet can impact the way that you sleep. Moreover, we will also be discussing the best practices when it comes to how you should structure your diet for optimal sleep. We will be discussing the top foods and drinks to eat or avoid in order to get the best sleep possible.

HOW YOUR NUTRIENTS AFFECT YOUR SLEEP

For the most part, people know that if they eat healthy and nutrient-rich foods, it will make their bodies function better. This is because the nutrients that come from food and get processed into your body's system can impact the chemical distribution of your body as well. If you are consistently eating healthy, then you are providing your brain with all of the chemicals that it needs to function the way that it should be functioning. This is also the reason why people who have poor dietary habits tend to have compromised cognitive function. Additionally, if you aren't eating well, then your brain won't have the chemical environment that it needs to promote good sleep. We've already talked about how your brain is one of the most important organs when it comes to determining the quality of your sleep. Aside from that, the recovery and recuperating processes that take place while you sleep are largely dependent on the quality of your diet. For example, we touched earlier on how muscle fibers are broken down after a hard training session and are typically repaired during sleep. Sleep, in itself, can't magically repair these broken muscle fibers. Your body needs protein and amino acids to ignite the process of rebuilding your muscles. So, if you aren't getting enough protein during the day, then you aren't getting all of the benefits of the restorative process that your body goes through while you sleep.

Aside from that, the food that you eat also has a huge impact on your body's natural circadian rhythm or body clock. Taking in substances like caffeine can dramatically alter your body's circadian rhythm, and that could lead to you having poor-quality sleep at night. It's also the same case with alcohol consumption.

THE BEST FOODS TO PROMOTE QUALITY SLEEP

For many years, sleep scientists, nutritionists, and other experts have conducted various research projects and experiments to determine how different foods can affect sleep. While much of the research does provide valuable data and information, it's not always conclusive. That's why continuous research is still being undertaken with regards to properties in food and how they affect a person's sleeping habits. It's also important to note that the nutrient profiles of certain foods aren't always consistent. For example, there are many different varieties of red grapes. Some of them have high levels of melatonin, which we all know by now is a sleep-inducing hormone. However, there are also some variants that have no melatonin at all. While research in this field is still ongoing, we've learned just enough to know about how certain foods can affect a person's sleep experience. Here are some of the best foods to promote the quality of your sleep.

Kiwi

This oval-shaped fruit is very commonly found in various countries all throughout the world, even though most people would typically associate it with New Zealand. Depending on where it grows, some varieties of kiwi can come in either green or golden colors. However, green kiwis tend to be the more common variant. The fruit itself possesses a lot of antioxidant properties, and researchers believe that this is the reason why many people tend to have improved sleep after kiwi consumption. However, no definitive studies have been able to determine the cause of such a phenomenon.

Tarragon

Tarragon is often used as a popular garnish for protein-rich dishes, especially in European countries. However, on its own, tarragon is also a very flavorful plant. It carries a lot of antioxidant properties while also supporting digestion. You can eat tarragon fresh as it is, or you can even turn it into a tea by boiling it in hot water for a few minutes and allowing it to steep. It's also a great option for people who want a pre-bedtime drink as it can help induce drowsiness.

Tart Cherry

Not to be confused with the more popular sweet cherry variant, tart cherries have a more sour flavor, as the name implies. They are also often referred to as sour cherries and are typically sold in bunches or in juice form. Tart cherries help regulate a body's circadian rhythm because they carry heavy doses of melatonin, which is a sleep-inducing hormone. One can reap the sleep benefits that come from eating cherries by drinking them in a juice form as well.

Kale

Kale is always touted as a superfood in fitness communities. Labeled the new spinach, it's a leafy vegetable that packs a punch by offering a lot of fiber, probiotics, and prebiotics. This makes it a digestion powerhouse. However, another thing that kale is rich in is melatonin. This is why eating raw kale for dinner would be a great way to prepare yourself to go to sleep early at night.

Rice

White rice, more specifically, is very good for helping people fall asleep. However, be very careful as even just one cup of white rice carries 250 calories with just 1 gram of fiber. It's also filled with a lot of sugar. So, just eat an appropriate amount of rice at night for dinner in order to help you fall asleep quicker.

Malted Milk

Malted milk, also called "nighttime milk," is a combination of traditional cow's milk with a specially formulated powder. This powder mostly consists of wheat flour, malted wheat, and malted barley. The most popular malted milk brand in the world is known as Horlick's. Again, just like the cherries, malted milk is filled with a lot of melatonin. This is because when cows are milked at night, their milk contains high levels of melatonin. These hormones are then transmitted to your body upon consumption.

Caffeine-Free Tea

If coffee is a great way to wake you up in the morning, caffeine-free tea is a great way for you to unwind and relax during the nighttime. You should opt for caffeine-free teas that won't stimulate your brain or give you any unwanted energy at night. Some examples of sleep-inducing teas include passionflower, chamomile, lemon balm, and hop teas.

Fatty Fish

Fatty fish such as tuna or salmon are also found to be good for promoting better sleep at night. This is because these kinds of fish are rich in omega-3 fatty acids and vitamin D. This protein is typically used for muscle building, joint strength, and improved immunity. An added benefit of eating these kinds of fish is the regulation of serotonin production in the body. Serotonin is another hormone that can contribute to higher-quality sleep.

Nuts

Nuts, just like kiwis, are loaded with antioxidants that could prove to be useful when promoting quality sleep. Aside from that, certain nut varieties like almonds, walnuts, cashews, and pistachios are known to carry healthy doses of melatonin. However, be very careful when eating nuts as they are loaded with calories and it can be very easy to overindulge in them.

THE WORST FOODS FOR QUALITY SLEEP

More than just pursuing foods and drinks that promote quality sleep, you should also look to actively avoid foods and drinks that could compromise the quality of your sleep. This is especially true for your nighttime consumption. Some foods are okay to be consumed within the day, and they won't typically affect the quality of your sleep as much. However, certain foods can keep you from falling asleep properly if you take them too late at night. Here are some of the worst possible foods and drinks for sleep.

Alcohol

Try to limit nightcaps as much as possible. We've already briefly touched on this in an earlier chapter, and it is true that alcohol helps people fall asleep faster. But we've also already learned that falling asleep earlier doesn't necessarily equate to a better quality of sleep. The most important aspect of sleep is going through the various sleep cycles properly so as to reap the benefits of each stage of the cycle. Unfortunately, alcohol has a way of deregulating the distribution of oxygen in your body. This can result in your inability to stay in a deep sleep for a longer period of time. Sometimes, if your body is too intoxicated, you may not even be able to enter a deep sleep to begin with.

Caffeine

This should practically go without saying, but you should always look to avoid drinking caffeine at night. However, the problem with this statement is that a lot of people think this purely means that they need to avoid drinking coffee at night. What they don't realize is that there are various other food and drink sources that carry caffeine as well. Most notably, dark chocolate is a common culprit. A lot of the commercial dark chocolate bars sold in stores carry heavy doses of caffeine. Aside from that, various teas such as the green and black variants carry a lot of caffeine as well. It's best to avoid these foods and drinks prior to bedtime.

Sugar

Sugar is one of the most influential culprits in determining your body's energy levels. You might have heard of the idea of people going into a sugar high and the corresponding crash that follows. This is because sugar acts as a primary source of energy for your body. Whenever you eat lots of simple sugar, your energy levels will spike abnormally, and this will result in hyperactivity in your brain. Sugar functions almost the same way a drug in terms of its level of stimulation. When that happens, it will make it harder for you to go to sleep.

Spicy, Gas-Inducing, and Acidic Foods

The last thing that you would want is to lie awake at night with severe discomfort in your stomach area as a result of acid reflux. Of course, this is on a case-to-case basis. Some people's bodies don't typically react to acidic or spicy foods so violently. Some people find it easy to go to sleep at night after consuming an entire pack of spicy noodles. However, for the most part, always try to avoid foods that can cause discomfort in your digestive system. The two most common culprits for this are spicy foods and acidic foods. When it comes to spicy foods, stay away from anything that has chili peppers in it. For acidic foods, try to stay away from acid-rich fruits like oranges or grapefruits. Also avoid food that makes you gassy. For example, if you're lactose-intolerant, then you need to avoid dairy as much as you can. This becomes all the more important at night. You don't want to be tossing and turning in your bed for hours because of that slice of pizza that you just couldn't resist.

GENERAL DIET TIPS FOR BETTER SLEEP

Eat More Tryptophan

Think back to a Thanksgiving dinner wherein you found yourself feeling really sleepy after devouring a lot of turkey. Some people might think that they were just drunk from overeating. But there might actually be another culprit that's inducing a sense of sleepiness in people during Thanksgiving, and that's tryptophan. This is an essential amino acid that is found in a variety of different foods like chicken, ground beef, milk, and turkey to name a few. The reason why tryptophan is often associated with inducing sleepiness is because it helps trigger the release of melatonin in your body. So, while turkey may not directly be the cause of you falling asleep earlier, the tryptophan that it carries certainly does.

Minimize Alcohol and Caffeine Intake Too Close to Bedtime

Earlier, we talked about the dangers of alcohol and caffeine when it comes to affecting your sleep. However, you shouldn't take that to mean that you're never allowed to take alcohol or caffeine ever again. It's really a matter of timing and moderation. When it comes to coffee, it's okay to have a cup or two earlier during the day. Ideally, you would take one in the morning and another one in the early afternoon at most. Anything more or later than that might affect your sleep. As far as alcohol is concerned, a glass of wine or a bottle of beer with your dinner shouldn't be a big deal. This is especially true if you're having dinner earlier at night. Heck, you can even get away with having a shot of whiskey, rum, or tequila if you want. Again, just make sure that you're limiting your intake to a reasonable amount and that you take these substances as early as you can.

Eat a Hearty Breakfast and a Conservative Dinner

You don't want to have your digestive system go into overdrive at night when you're supposed to be relaxing and winding down. This is why it wouldn't be an idea to completely stuff yourself with food at night. As much as possible, you want to minimize your food intake at night so that your body won't be primed to exert a lot of energy to process your food intake. There's an old saying that goes, "Breakfast like a king and dinner like a pauper." You should try to adopt that strategy if you're looking to sleep better at night. Aside from that, limiting your food intake at night may even help you shed some unwanted pounds.

Review Your Meds

Maintenance meds are fine. In most cases, they're even necessary. However, you should pay closer attention to the ingredients in these meds of yours. Some medicines and supplements out there are filled with caffeine. You may not be drinking coffee, but you're still getting that same buzz by taking in a tablet of your maintenance meds. Again, if this is the case, you don't have to give up your meds entirely just so you can have better sleep. Just try to take any caffeinated meds or supplements earlier within the day. Most of the time, medications for headaches and colds might be dosed with a little bit of caffeine. Make sure to consult your doctor for further clarification.

Don't Smoke Late at Night

Smoking is bad for you, and it's a habit that you should try to quit altogether if you engage in it regularly. However, if you must smoke, then at least try to limit your smoking late at night. Research suggests that nicotine can have a huge impact on your circadian rhythm. Nicotine is an active ingredient in cigarettes that is responsible for making smoking so addicting. Aside from that, smoking also has a way of compromising one's capacity to take in more oxygen. We've already talked about how important it is for the body to take in oxygen while sleeping. Failing to regulate the body's oxygen intake would result in one's inability to enter into deeper stages of sleep.

Be Careful When Using Sleeping Pills

There's a good and bad side to sleeping pills, and that's why you want to be as careful as possible if you're ever taking them consistently. Sure, many doctors will assign patients sleeping pills as a solution for issues like insomnia. In fact, the rate at which people consume sleeping pills nowadays is alarmingly high. There's nothing inherently wrong with sleeping pills as they are medically demonstrated to help people sleep better. If you use them correctly, then they can help you develop better sleeping habits. However, there are cases wherein people abuse the use of sleeping pills, and this can cause more serious problems down the line. If you decide on using them for yourself, make sure that you are under the guided supervision of a doctor. These drugs also tend to be very addictive and are never designed for long-term use.

Stay Hydrated

Lastly, the last thing you want to remember when it comes to your diet is to drink more water. You may not think that staying hydrated could affect your sleep so much, but it actually does. Drinking too much water before bedtime may cause you to wake up in the middle of the night for a bathroom break, so avoid drinking too much liquids so close to bedtime. However, you don't want to go to bed dehydrated either. This is why it's important for you to stay hydrated all throughout the day. If you're not getting enough water, then your mouth and nasal passages can become dry. This can lead to snoring and could potentially pull you out of your deep sleep prematurely.

PERSONAL STORY

I must confess that situations like this have happened to me quite a few times already. One time, I decided that I would put a lot of effort into my meal because I was in the mood for something special. I decided on Asian hot pot, since it can be hard to go wrong with that. For anyone who isn't aware of what Asian hot pot is, it's essentially a dish that originated in the oriental parts of the continent. You place a huge pot on top of a portable gas stove and fill it with broth. Then, you need to bring the broth to a light simmer before dumping in loads of different fresh ingredients. People tend to take liberties when deciding on what ingredients to add. For the most part, you want fresh ingredients like vegetables, spices, and meats that will make the broth much more flavorful. You can add stuff like carrots, spring onions, cabbages, turnips, corn, shrimps, beef, chicken, and whatnot. It's mostly made to function like an interactive meal wherein people at the table get to scoop up the parts of the broth that they want the most.

This one time, after preparing all of the ingredients, thawing the meats, and washing the vegetables, the meal was finally ready at around 9 p.m. I was preparing a lot of ingredients, and that's why it took a while for the meal to be ready. We ended up finishing our dinner at around 11 p.m. This is much later than most people's usual dinner time. However, even though we ate our dinner a little later that night, we still decided to go to bed at our regular 12:30 a.m. bedtime. I can't tell you how much time on the clock went by with me just tossing and turning in my bed trying to go to sleep. I was struggling to relax myself, but my stomach just felt so full and uncomfortable from such a big and savory meal. I didn't give my tummy enough time to completely process and digest everything. What ended up happening was my partner and I got up and ended up just talking for another hour while waiting for our stomachs to completely digest everything.

Essentially, the point is to always be mindful of how your food affects your body, especially when it comes to sleeping.

7

POSITION YOURSELF

ou may not think that the position in which you sleep has much impact on the quality of your sleep. After all, as long as you're getting some rest, what difference does it make if you're in one position or the other? Unfortunately, the answer to that question is a bit more complicated than you might think. In this chapter, we are going to talk more about how your sleeping position affects your sleep, the consequences of getting into certain positions, and how you can figure out your own optimal position for sleeping at night.

We've already talked exhaustively about the numerous factors that could affect a person's ability to fall asleep and stay asleep. We know that environmental factors, daily habits, and mental health have a lot to do with it. However, we haven't really discussed how sleeping position can also be a big factor as well. Earlier, when we were talking about pillows and mattresses, we briefly touched on the idea of different sleeping positions. Of course, not everyone sleeps the same way. Heck, you might even sleep in a different position on a night-to-night basis. The point here is that none of us ever really pay as much attention to our sleeping positions as we should. Hopefully, after going through this chapter, you will realize that there is so much more to your sleeping position than you may have initially thought.

WHAT YOUR SLEEPING POSITION DOES TO YOUR SPINE

You still probably remember being a child and being told by a parent or a teacher to sit or stand up straight because it would be good for your posture. Whenever you were slouching while you walked or when you were seated, a grown-up would be quick to tell you to straighten your spine because better posture meant better spinal health and strength. Eventually, over time, you would hear these voices in your head reminding you to adopt better posture whenever you would sink down into a slouch. For the most part, these are the positions that we associate with developing better posture. However, there is one more position that the adults might not have taught you about when you were younger, a position that's absolutely crucial for promoting spinal health as well. That's your sleeping position.

Depending on how you position your body at night when you sleep, your posture can have significant negative effects on the strength, stability, and overall health of your spine. On top of that, when you take into consideration that the spine is a chain that connects to other major parts of your body, that means that your sleeping position can affect the way that your entire body functions as well. Keep in mind that whatever position you fall asleep with is likely one that you will stay in for hours on end. Of course, you may go through a few tosses and turns at night. But for the most part, you sustain these positions for a long period of time. When you put your body in a skewed, twisted, or crooked position that's awkward and uncomfortable, it can create a lot of tension and stress on your back. Remember that the whole point of sleep is to relieve yourself of any stress so that you can regain the energy that you need to face the next day. If you sleep in a compromised position, then your body wouldn't be able to go through an optimal rejuvenation process.

You may have already experienced waking up from a deep slumber with an annoying crick in your neck or a lingering soreness at the base of your spine. Sometimes, you might even find yourself waking up in the middle of the night because your limbs have fallen asleep as a result of your blood circulation being compromised. Whatever the case, if you are waking up feeling uncomfortable or in pain, then your sleeping position is the likely culprit.

The part of your body that your sleeping posture can influence the most is your spine. As much as possible, you want to keep your spine in a fully aligned and relaxed position. Distribute weight as evenly as possible so that no one particular region or area of your spine is bearing most of the load while you sleep. For example, if you position your pillows in such a way that your pillow is too tall, then that might create a lot of tension on your shoulders. You are essentially placing yourself in a hunched position the same way that you would when you are slouched over a desk. If your pillow is too short, then you could cause your neck to go into a hyper-extended position wherein the curve of your neck is far too extreme. This can cause severe stress and pressure on your neck muscles. That's just one example of how your sleeping position can affect your body, and that's just the neck we're talking about. In the latter parts of this chapter, we will go over various sleeping positions and the specific impact that each of them has on your body.

HOW YOUR SLEEPING POSTURE IMPACTS YOUR HEALTH

There's this urban legend that says that you spend around a third of your life in bed; however, there aren't any definitive studies that can corroborate this statement. Even then, we all know that we spend a huge chunk of our time asleep in bed. Given that, shouldn't we be paying closer attention to the way that we position ourselves? The way that you position your body isn't just a matter of comfort. It's also about making sure that you're staying healthy. For example, many people seem to find it comfortable to go to sleep in a fetal position. But a lot of them don't know that this position lessens the likelihood of developing back problems. Interestingly enough, people who sleep in the fetal position are also less likely to get Alzheimer's or Parkinson's disease (Moghim, 2020). The point here is that the masses don't really comprehend just how impactful their sleeping position can be in terms of their health.

Yes, sleep is essential to you having the energy to be a productive employee at work or student at school in order to complete tasks. You need sleep in order to be motivated and driven to make something of yourself. In this part of the chapter, we will go over some of the most common sleeping positions and what kind of impact they can have on your overall health and wellness.

Fetal Position

The fetal position is when you sleep on your side with your legs pulled up towards your torso. It's estimated that roughly around 40% of human beings sleep in this position. The reason why people tend to naturally deviate towards this position is because it provides optimal comfort and alignment for the spine. Research has shown that getting into such a position is also good for flushing out toxins in the brain. This is why, as we mentioned earlier, getting into a fetal position decreases the likelihood of developing neurological illnesses like Parkinson's or Alzheimer's disease. Research also suggests that the fetal position is a good option for pregnant women because it improves the circulation for the mother and the child. Some people position a pillow in between their knees while in a fetal position to promote better blood flow and to relieve pressure. Aside from that, another benefit of sleeping in the fetal position (and any other kind of position that has you sleeping on your side) is that it's good for people who have a tendency to snore.

However, it's not all good when it comes to the fetal position. There are certain caveats as well. One major disadvantage of sleeping on your side (not just the fetal position) is that one side of your face is in direct contact with the pillow. Pressing your face down on a surface like this for prolonged periods can cause the development of wrinkles on the face. Aside from that, women may be prone to have their breasts sag over time because of how the breast stretches while lying down on one's side. However, there are no definitive studies that can render this as conclusive.

Log Position

The log position is another sleeping position that has you lying down on your side. However, instead of curling yourself up like a fetus, the log position has your body almost perfectly straight... much like a log. Approximately around 15% of people in the world sleep in a log position with their arms and legs completely extended towards the bottom of the bed. The reason this position is relatively healthy is because it maintains a neutral spine. This means that there isn't any unnecessary pressure or torque on the spine while you sleep.

However, all of the previously mentioned disadvantages of sleeping on one's side still apply to the log position as well.

Spooning Position

The last side-sleeping position that we will be discussing here is one that is commonly conducted by couples who sleep in the same bed together. This is often referred to as the "spooning position," wherein two people are locked in a half embrace while they sleep. The way that the spooning position works is that both people are sleeping on their sides while facing the same direction. The person in the back holds the front person close to their body. This kind of position certainly has its fair share of pros and cons.

For the first con, people are more likely to wake up from this position, especially when your partner jostles about at night. Another problem is when the back partner has their arm under the front partner, it may fall asleep due to the lack of blood circulation. This can cause them to wake up in the middle of the night due to the discomfort.

The pros include that cuddling with a partner triggers the release of oxytocin. This is also known as a "happy hormone" and is responsible for creating a bond between two people. This hormone is also effective at fighting off stress, which we all know is one of the biggest impediments to quality sleep at night.

Freefall Position

A freefall position is one that has you sleeping on your stomach with your head pointed towards one side. An estimated 7% of people sleep on their stomachs this way, and it's not the most optimal sleeping position. Putting yourself in a freefall position is not good for your neck and back. This is because rotating your head towards the side in such a manner prevents your neck and spine from having a neutral alignment.

There are certain upsides to having such a position such as eliminating snoring and sleep apnea. However, the cons vastly outweigh the pros in this instance. There's just too much tension and pressure that's generated around the neck and spine because of the negative curvature. This position is also likely to have you tossing and turning while you sleep, which could keep you from entering the deeper stages of sleep.

Starfish Position

The starfish position is also a relatively popular sleeping position with around 8% of people using it consistently. With the starfish position, people lie down on their backs with their arms and legs splayed out in different directions, almost like a starfish. Typically, this kind of position only works on a big bed with ample space. While this position isn't going to be as bad for your spine as sleeping on your stomach, it's still not an optimal sleeping position. This is because lying down on your back for prolonged periods could create lots of tension on your lower spine. Aside from that, you are more prone to snoring and sleep apnea when you are lying down on your back.

Soldier Position

The soldier sleeping position also has you lying down on your back, but with your arms resting against the sides of your body. Like the starfish position, an estimated 8% of people sleep like this. The soldier position carries a lot of the negatives of the starfish position, such as increased pressure on the lower back and increased likelihood of sleep apnea and snoring. However, it is still much better for your spine than sleeping on your stomach.

HOW TO CHANGE YOUR SLEEPING POSTURE

If you find that your sleeping position is less than optimal, then you may want to consider changing it. For example, if you experience lower back soreness, it may be because you constantly sleep facing up. So, you've decided that you want to try sleeping on your side, but you don't exactly know how to go about it. After all, so many people think that sleeping posture is a completely natural thing that people just fall into and can't change. However, that isn't necessarily true. Yes, you can grow accustomed to a certain sleeping position over time the more that you practice it. But it doesn't always have to be a permanent situation. You can actively change your sleeping position into something that seems more natural over time with a little effort. It might feel a little awkward at first, but if changing your position means lessening your neck or back pain, then it's definitely going to be worth it.

Before we move into discussing *how* you can change your sleeping position, it's important that you be sure about what you're doing. Yes, getting into a certain position might alleviate your back pain or lessen the chances of you developing wrinkles on your face. However, at the end of the day, the goal is to promote optimal sleep. If your position is getting in the way of you getting a good night's sleep, then you may want to rethink your plan here. It's important that you understand that there are certain trade-offs for any choice that you make, and you just have to be sure about it. With that said, here are a few things that you can try to alter your sleeping position.

1. Make use of your pillows. Experiment with how your pillows are positioned on your bed. Earlier, we talked about how different pillows suit different sleeping types. Feel free to refer to that chapter for a refresher. More than just the pillow type, you may want to experiment how the pillows are laid out on your bed as well. This can take a little experimentation, but you'll eventually settle on a layout that best suits you.

2. Try different mattresses. There are some high-end mattresses these days that offer a great deal of adjustability. If you're someone who likes to sleep on your back but you also want to elevate your legs, then certain mattresses will allow you to get into such a position. Other mattresses are better adjusted for people who sleep on their sides or stomachs. You can pay a visit to a local mattress store to see what they have to offer.

3. Use a tennis ball. One cheap hack that you can use is to sew a tennis ball onto the side of your shirt that you don't want to sleep on. That way, when you roll over to that side, the tennis ball will make it uncomfortable for you and will force you to return to your ideal position. You may find yourself waking up in the middle of the night a lot at first. But it's a solid temporary solution as you're trying to acclimate yourself to a new position.

PERSONAL STORY

I used to sleep really weirdly. It was just this random tic that I had every night before going to bed. Somehow, as I readied my body for sleeping, I always wanted to position my right arm in such a way that it was fully extended towards the side. Otherwise, things just felt really off and uncomfortable for me. I found it difficult to go to sleep if I were in any other kind of position. At the time, I considered it completely normal and I didn't think much of it. It just happened to be the way that I wanted to sleep, and I stuck to it. Aside from that, I would position my left palm so that it was resting directly on my stomach. Again, it was another one of those things wherein, if it were in any other position, I wouldn't be comfortable. It would have been impossible for me to go to sleep and that would render me drowsy and groggy at work. This was definitely not an option as I always wanted to be performing at my best when it came to office work.

Anyway, there was one day wherein I was having a random conversation with a few of my work colleagues and we chanced upon the topic of sleeping positions. I shared to them what my optimal sleeping position was and I found myself thinking that it was kind of weird that I always needed to get into such a position to fall asleep. As I listened to my colleagues share their personal experiences and positions when falling asleep, I found it even weirder. I had one coworker who told me that she liked to sleep with her entire body facing downward. My first thought was that putting myself in that kind of position would make it difficult for me to breathe. Aside from that, she even admitted that sleeping in that kind of position had given her back pain. However, since she was convinced that it was the only way that she could fall asleep at night, she just kept on doing it.

This piqued my interest about sleep positions even further and I decided to do a little digging around online. It was only then that I found out that my position of having to extend my right arm and rest my left palm on my stomach didn't really matter. In fact, it was kind of weird that I was so obsessive about getting into that kind of position to begin with. The science taught me that I was being inefficient and that forcing myself to get into such a position prior to bed was counterproductive to what I was trying to achieve. My research led to me abandoning my old sleeping positions that I had grown so attached to. At first, I was somewhat skeptical, and I still thought that I would sleep better if I stuck with my old sleeping position. But after the first few nights, I was still sleeping fine. In fact, I was sleeping better now that I had adopted more optimal positions for sleep.

8

A CLEAR MIND

e've finally reached the end of the book, and for this last chapter, we're going to tackle one of the most important aspects of getting a good night's sleep: your mind. Ultimately, your mind can either be your greatest threat or closest ally when it comes to getting quality sleep at night. If your mind is constantly running and ruminating about the most random things at night, then this might keep you from getting some much-needed shuteye. However, if you have a clear and calm mind that is able to relax itself easily, then the process of going to sleep will be much simpler.

Before we get deeper into this chapter, it's important to stress that if you're experiencing any mental health issues, it would be best for you to seek the professional advice and treatment of a licensed expert. This book is not a solution to mental health problems. Mental health is a serious matter that needs to be treated by dedicated professionals who are deeply immersed in this field. Rather, what this final chapter will seek to provide is further insight into simple hacks and approaches on how you can restore your mind to a more restful and stress-free state. Again, this shouldn't serve as an alternative to proper treatment for serious mental health.

WHAT KEEPS YOU UP AT NIGHT?

The truth is that there is still so much to be learned about the connections between mental health and sleep. Even now, experts and scientists are conducting exhaustive research into the matter. It's an incredibly complex topic that has to take into consideration so many different factors and variables. Given that, we know so much more now about the connections between sleep and mental activity. And it's important that you understand how both of these concepts impact one another so that you gain better control over them.

As you have already learned when we were talking about sleep stages and sleep cycles, your brain activity can fluctuate while you sleep. It can be somewhat active when you're awake as it gradually dips into REM wherein your brain will pick up energy once again. However, for the restorative process of sleep, your brain needs to slow down significantly. This is the only way you can really get the benefits of the deep sleep stage. This is why it's hard for people to feel like they're sleeping well when they're dealing with mental issues. These mental issues can be taking up too much space in the mind, and they can prevent the brain from winding down. It's constantly engaged in a state of stimulation because these negative ideas and concepts demand their attention.

Of course, it's a different situation for everyone. Some of us may be dealing with minor challenges or struggles in life that are stressing us out. For the most part, the stress that comes with these rough patches is manageable and can be treated fairly quickly. However, there are also some people who might be dealing with more serious personal issues that require a more experienced and dedicated kind of treatment. If you feel like your mental problems are keeping you from getting quality sleep, then you may want to consider seeing a licensed professional for treatment. In particular, cognitive behavioral therapy (CBT) is a popular form of counseling that's often referred to as talk therapy. Through CBT, you can discuss your issues with a licensed expert, and they would be in the best position to help you manage your problems more methodically and scientifically. Many people who struggle with insomnia and find themselves incapable of treating their sleep issues on their own often resort to CBT as an alternative treatment. It has a good track record in alleviating the sleeping problems of people who have certain mental health issues.

HOW STRESS AFFECTS YOUR SLEEP

Insomnia is more common than you might think. In fact, roughly anywhere between 10 to 30% of adults have insomnia (Bhaskar et al., 2016). Also, if you know someone who's dealing with insomnia, more often than not, that condition is being caused by stress. It doesn't matter how nice your sleeping environment is or how conducive your bed is for actual sleep. If you're dealing with stress, it can really compromise your ability to get a good night's sleep. People with insomnia typically have trouble sleeping at least three times a week for a period of around three months. There are many possible stressors that can contribute to the development of chronic insomnia, such as:

- sudden loss of a loved one

- illness or injury
- professional dissatisfaction
- financial difficulties
- relationship problems
- dramatic life changes, etc.

Of course, this isn't to say that everyone who is stressed is automatically going to experience insomnia. After all, everyone experiences stress to a certain extent. It's just that people who aren't able to manage their stress effectively tend to end up compromising the quality of their sleep as a result. This is especially true for people who are suffering from anxiety or some other kind of mental health disorder. The most difficult part about developing insomnia as a result of stress is that the symptoms only compound the problem even further. We already talked about how a lack of sleep can gradually eat away at a person's mental stability. More than that, here are other symptoms that you might experience as a result of chronic insomnia:

- fatigue
- difficulty focusing or concentrating
- compromised social performance
- irritability and mood swings
- hyperactivity
- irrationality
- decreased motivation
- increased likelihood for mistakes and accidents

It can be very difficult to pinpoint what a person's specific stressors are because it's really a different case from person to person. For example, a particular problem that might be incredibly stressful for person A may not necessarily have the same effects on person B. This is why addressing mental health issues like this can be really tricky and may sometimes necessitate the intervention of a professional. However, before resorting to one's professional advice and guidance, it wouldn't hurt to practice a few exercises of your own in order to induce a sense of calm and relaxation within yourself.

WHAT TO DO IF YOUR MIND IS RACING

One common symptom of insomnia is when people find their brains becoming hyperactive in the middle of the night. No matter how hard they try, they can't just seem to drift off into dreamland. They can close their eyes by making use of sleep masks, but it still doesn't help them much. Their mind is just too active, and it's displaying all sorts of different pictures in their head. A lot of the time, all of this hyperactivity is merely a manifestation of daily stressors. It's the things that you keep at the back of your mind which are actually calling for your attention.

For example, you might have marital problems. You may be going through financial troubles. Things might not be going so well at work. Again, it could be for a variety of different reasons. Sometimes, it may even be a combination of different problems put together. It can be really irritating when all you want to do is fall asleep, but your mind just refuses to cooperate. Fortunately, there is a relatively quick fix for this, especially if your issues aren't so deep-seated. We've already talked about how a hyperactive mind can often be a result of certain anxieties or stressors in your life. Obviously, if you are able to address those stressors, then that would be the best course of action. You are addressing the root of the problem. But if you're looking for quicker fixes that you can employ while you're already in bed, then here are a few things that you can try out:

- Get out of bed and find another place to relax.
- Do mindful meditation and breathing exercises.
- Address your thoughts and immediately let them go.
- Count your blessings and remind yourself of what you're grateful for.
- Engage in a sensory practice by paying closer attention to all your senses.

Sometimes, one of the best ways to really calm your mind would be to engage in some kind of sensory practice. This will again enforce the idea of mindfulness, and it will help generate a sense of calm within yourself. Take note that you have five senses. You don't necessarily have to practice every single one, but engaging in one or two might help induce a sense of calm.

Sight

When you want to practice your sense of sight, make sure to avoid blue light as much as possible. Keep the lighting in your space dim and warm so that you aren't activating your brain too much. Then, try to browse through calming photos of nature or abstract colors that will help you forget about your worries temporarily. Go for images that are peaceful to you. Again, what constitutes as peaceful can vary from person to person.

Smell

It always helps to light a candle in your room to induce a sense of calm. Ideally, you want to go for softer and more subtle scents like lavender or sandalwood. These are good, calming aromas that can really help you steady your mind.

Aside from candles, you can also make use of essential oil diffusers. Focus on the smell and try to think about how these scents make you feel. Allow the scents to completely take over your senses.

Touch

We've already covered the basics of your sleeping environment in an earlier chapter, so there's no need to go too in depth here. Just as a refresher, you should surround yourself with a proper mattress, pillow, and bedsheet that are suitable to your sleeping preferences. Aside from that, you can opt to take a warm bath or have a light stretch to help calm you down a bit.

Taste

We've already discussed that it wouldn't be wise for you to be having too much food or drinks immediately before going to bed. However, if you have a hyperactive mind, you may consider getting a light sleep-friendly snack or a cup of caffeine-free tea that will help you sleep.

Sound

When it comes to sound, you don't want anything that is too disruptive or energetic. So, avoid listening to music that hypes you up. Instead, opt for music that is calming and relaxing. Consider going for instrumental music or soft classical music. If you're not big on music, you can also try to focus on white noise from falling rain, running AC units or electric fans, or even the chirping of crickets. Focus on these natural sounds and allow them to calm you down.

POSITIVE THOUGHTS TO THINK ABOUT BEFORE BED

Negative energy can really take away from the quality of your sleep. When you're constantly dwelling on the things that stress you out, then you're holding on to a lot of negative energy. None of this is good for sleep, and you should try to train your mind to adopt more positive thoughts while you sleep. If you struggle with conjuring up this positive energy on your own, then there are a few mental exercises that you may want to consider putting yourself through every night before bed. More than just helping you sleep at night, having an optimistic and positive disposition will improve the quality of your life in other ways as well. It will allow you to be more sociable, and it will give you resilience and motivation to tackle life's challenges.

Focus on Your Favorite Part of Your Day

One great way to practice gratitude and humility is to always remind yourself of just how good you have it in life. Of course, that isn't to say that you have a perfect life and that you don't have any problems. It's just a matter of keeping things in perspective. Rather than going to bed at night dwelling on all the bad things that are going on, try to focus and center your mind around the good. This can be an incredibly therapeutic activity, and it can be particularly useful at putting you into the proper mood for going to sleep.

Think back to that one moment during your day when you felt incredibly happy or grateful to be alive. Maybe it was a hug that a loved one gave you. Maybe your boss gave you a compliment over the work that you've done. Maybe you really enjoyed that slice of pizza that you had for lunch.

Whatever it is, remind yourself of the elation that you felt in that moment and focus on it. Try to simulate that feeling again as you prepare your mind and body for sleep.

Picture the Most Beautiful Place You Can Possibly Imagine

No, this isn't an excuse for you to grab your phone and open up your Instagram. Just lie down in bed and use the screen that exists inside of your mind. Picture the most beautiful place that you could possibly imagine in your own head. This place could either be real or fictitious. It doesn't really matter as long as it's a place that gives you a sense of calm and happiness. For some, it could be the image of a beach with clear blue skies and a bright yellow sun whose rays are shimmering in the water. For others, it could be in a quiet museum in the middle of France, surrounded by the greatest paintings the world has ever known. Others might find happiness in imagining a vast meadow with a soft breeze blowing through the surrounding trees. It could be absolutely anything that sparks a sense of joy and wonder in your heart.

Give Yourself Positive Affirmations

Positive affirmations are always great, even for times wherein you're not trying to fall asleep. However, it can feel really good to go to sleep at night knowing that you believe in yourself and that you're choosing to stay positive despite everything that life is throwing your way. Again, when you're struggling to go to sleep at night, it's usually because your mind is dwelling on things that are stressing you out. The natural way of counteracting that would be to dwell on positive things about yourself. And the best thing about positive affirmations is that they can be anything that you want them to be. The only important thing here is that you genuinely believe it and that it makes you feel happy. Here are a few examples of positive affirmations:

- "I am happy with where I am at in life."
- "I choose to be content with the life that I have."
- "I have what it takes to tackle the challenges that are in front of me."
- "I am capable of great things."
- "I can do anything I set my mind to."

Focus on Nothing but Your Breathing

We've already talked about how oxygen is important for sleep. Feel free to go back to the earlier chapter wherein we discussed a breathing exercise that you can practice at night to help you go to sleep.

Focus on Something You're Excited About

This might seem counterproductive to some people given that you may not want your brain to get hyped up or excited about something. However, there's also something incredibly calming about knowing that there are great things that lie ahead for you in the future. It helps ease any sense of anxiety or uncertainty that you may have. Rather than worrying about what future problems await you in the future, focus on the things that you know make you feel happy and excited about.

Be Okay With Not Falling Asleep Right Away

Sometimes, even the mere desire to fall asleep right away is what is causing you so much stress. For instance, you know that you have a big presentation coming up at work for the next day. So, you end up placing yourself under a lot of pressure to go to sleep early. You know that you need all the energy and focus you can get. This is why you try your best to get as much sleep as you can. However, despite your best intentions, you find yourself tossing and turning at night, unable to fall asleep. You keep running the numbers through your mind as you try to figure out how much sleep you could still possibly get. You're creating more and more pressure for yourself to fall asleep, and this is counterproductive to what you want to achieve.

So, instead of trying to fight your insomnia, try to be okay with it. Try to accept it. Be okay with not falling asleep right away. When you accept that this is what is happening to you, you will be surprised at how incredibly calming it can be. As a result, you will find it a lot easier to fall asleep right after.

EXERCISES TO TRY BEFORE BED

In an earlier chapter, we talked about the 4-7-8 breathing exercise that you could use as a tool to relax and prepare yourself for sleep. We've also talked about certain stretches and poses that you could put yourself in to prime your body for sleeping earlier and better. However, there are also other exercises that you can try to prepare yourself for bed. These exercises are more designed to help you achieve mental calm and relaxation. They're relatively simple to perform, and there's really nothing to lose in trying them out when you constantly suffer from going to sleep early.

Body Scan

Think of a body scan as your way of actively checking up on the various parts of your body. It's a great meditative exercise that is designed to promote mindfulness and awareness over your own body. It's also a great way to help you relax yourself as you prepare for bed. Perform the following steps to execute a full body scan:

1. When lying down in bed, take a few deep breaths using the 4-7-8 breathing technique. This will help put you into a more relaxed state.
2. As you continue your breathing, bring your attention to your feet. Start at the very tip of your toes and work your way down all the way to your heels.
3. Notice if there is any tightness, soreness, or tension in that part of the body.
4. If you feel tension, then focus all of your energy on that area and channel your breath towards that region. Visualize the tension leaving that part of your body with every exhale.
5. When you feel like you've let go of that tension, move on from your feet and proceed to your calf muscles.
6. Repeat the process of mindfulness and visualization there. Look for any tense or hot spots and focus your energies on releasing yourself from such tension.
7. Perform this exercise for every single part of your body until you reach the top of your head.

Muscle Relaxation

Another exercise you can use to prepare for bedtime is the progressive muscle relaxation technique. Essentially, it serves the same purpose as the body scan wherein it allows you to generate more awareness over your body. It also involves you actively releasing tension from your muscles.

But more than that, this exercise is geared towards really relaxing your muscles and allowing them to be in their most inactive states. Many people will have different approaches to the muscle relaxation technique, and that's fine. You can even try to figure out a path of your own to see which one would work best for you.

1. Start the exercise by lying down in bed and doing a quick mental recall of all the major muscle groups in your body. This can include your hands, forearms, upper arms, back, chest, abdomen, hips, thighs, calves, feet, and others. Again, it's up to you.
2. Focus on just one muscle group first. Let's say that you're choosing a top-down approach and you're starting with your shoulders.
3. Breathe in deeply and while doing so, engage your shoulder muscles to create tension for around five to 10 seconds.
4. As you breathe out, let go of the tension in that muscle group.
5. Take around 10 to 20 seconds as you try to relax before moving on to another muscle group and repeating the process until you cover your entire body or until you fall asleep.

Biofeedback

The last exercise you can try might be a little more complicated because it requires a bit of technological assistance. With biofeedback, by making use of electronic devices, you are able to monitor various body signals that are connected to sleeping such as heart rate, oxygen levels, and body temperature. From this data, you would be able to understand the quality of your sleep better and you would also be in an optimal position to correct any problems in real time.

For example, you may be struggling with going to sleep. One glance at your smartwatch with a sleep tracker will tell you that your heart rate is too high and is not in the optimal range for sleeping. This could be a result of anxious thoughts about an upcoming project or challenge in your life. Then, you could adjust by employing an anti-anxiety breathing technique or meditation exercise that could lower your heart rate. A biofeedback tool might also be able to tell you that your body temperature is still too high to allow you to sleep comfortably. So, you could adjust by turning the thermostat of your AC down a little so that your body will cool down as well.

PERSONAL STORY

For this final chapter's personal anecdote, I am sure that a lot of people will have also experienced this in the past in some shape or form. Personally, I have found myself staying awake at night as a result of financial stress and personal heartbreak on a number of occasions.

There was a time wherein my sister had serious financial troubles. She was buried underneath piles of debt, and it was becoming too much for her to handle all by herself. Being her sibling, I decided to put a pause on my own personal dreams and goals for a while so that I could devote some of my resources to helping her out. I told my sister that I would help tackle some of her payments. At that time, she was a single mother of two kids, and she really didn't have anyone else that she could rely on. No one had her back and I felt obligated to try my best to alleviate her troubles.

Things went fine at first, but they didn't stay that way. Her debt troubles just kept on growing, and I had to increase my efforts the more we went along. I barely had enough extra money for myself. I couldn't even afford to hang out with my friends and I was struggling to pay my own bills. This went on for around two years, and it deeply troubled me. I was under a lot of stress and pressure on behalf of my sister. Throughout those two years, I had trouble going to sleep at night. I would always lie in bed thinking about what it would be like to go bankrupt. I spent so many hours lying awake, trying to comprehend the mountain of debt that still stood in our way. Truthfully, I didn't even realize just how big of a toll this financial problem was taking on my mental and physical health.

Aside from financial woes, I've also had my fair share of heartbreaks. Unfortunately, no matter how hard you try, some relationships just don't work out. It's not necessarily because you don't love the other person. A lot of the time, a relationship can still end even when two people are deeply in love with one another. Unfortunately, love alone is never enough to sustain a relationship, and that's what makes these breakups even harder to deal with. The thought of ending a relationship and the pain that came along with it made me feel so down and restless for many nights. Of course, the natural thoughts of regrets and obsessions over how I possibly could have done things better continuously plagued my mind. I also spent many nights replaying the happiest moments of our relationship as I struggled to keep a hold of those memories. There were so many conversations and plans that all went down the drain with the breakup, and I was struggling to let them go. More than anything, what kept me up at night was really the anxiety and fear of having to face a future without the person that I thought I would be spending the rest of my life with. There's a different kind of pain that's associated with that experience, and it's not one that's easy to confront or deal with. It's the kind of pain that just demands to be felt, and it doesn't go away too easily. I've literally cried myself to sleep on numerous occasions, and my pillowcase would be moist with tears by the time I fall asleep.

What I'm trying to say here is that we are all human beings. As human beings, we are all inclined to have feelings and it's not always possible for us to switch our emotions off. Anxieties can creep in whether we invite them or not. This is why it's very important that we make conscious efforts to really address the negativity that may linger in our minds. We need to establish a sense of control over these situations so that they don't take control of us.

AFTERWORD

We've finally reached the end of the book, and it's possible that you may be feeling a little overwhelmed. Who would have known that there's so much you need to be mindful of when you go to sleep at night? In this book, we talked about why sleep is important and the science behind how it affects your body. We've also talked about the dangers of practicing poor sleeping habits and how they could potentially compromise your quality of life. If you're someone who experiences sleeping problems, then you now have further insight into what might be causing these problems to begin with. Moreover, you may also have more knowledge on how you can potentially combat the root causes of your sleeping woes so that you can get better sleep at night.

We've learned about the various techniques that you can employ to promote better sleep. You now know that diet can play a huge part in determining how well you sleep at night. You also now know that the way that your bedroom is structured and designed can significantly impact your sleeping experience. We've discussed the science behind choosing pillows, mattresses, lights, and even sleeping positions that could promote optimal sleep. We've touched on the different sleep stages and the roles that they play in keeping your body healthy and fit.

Most importantly, you should have developed a better relationship with your sleeping habits by now. Sleep isn't just something that you can afford to approach passively. It's something that you need to be mindful of because of how significant a role that it plays in shaping your life. By forging a better relationship with your sleeping habits, you will give your body the rest and rejuvenation that it needs to be ready to face the world every single day.

REFERENCES

Bennett, J. (2019, November 14). *How to light your home for the best sleep ever*. Better Homes & Gardens. https://www.b-hg.com/home-improvement/lighting/planning/light-for-best-sleep/

Bhaskar, S., Hemavathy, D., & Prasad, S. (2016). Prevalence of chronic insomnia in adult patients and its correlation with medical comorbidities. *Journal of Family Medicine and Primary Care, 5*(4), 780. https://doi.org/10.4103/2249-4863.201153

Blaivas, A., Turley, R., & Pierce-Smith, D. (2020). *Sleep deprivation*. Cedars-Sinai. https://www.cedars-sinai.org/health-library/diseases-and-conditions/s/sleep-deprivation.html

Block, L. (2021, June 28). *How to choose a mattress—guide to your best night's sleep*. Sleepopolis. https://sleepopolis.-com/guides/how-to-choose-a-mattress/

Bowling, N. (2016, May 4). *Aerobic vs. anaerobic: What's best for weight loss?* (P. Pletcher, Ed.). Healthline. https://www.healthline.com/health/fitness-exercise/aerobic-vs-anaerobic#The-science-behind-aerobic-vs.-anaerobic

Cordeiro, B. (2014, April). *8 healthy sleep habits*. MD Anderson Cancer Center. https://www.mdanderson-.org/publications/focused-on-health/healthy-sleep-habits.h13-1589046.html

Davis, C. P. (2021, May 17). *Sleep: What are the best sleeping positions?* OnHealth; OnHealth. https://www.onhealth.-com/content/1/best_sleeping_positions_sleep

DiGiulio, S. (2017a, October 9). *What happens in your body and brain while you sleep*. NBC News; NBC News. https://www.n-bcnews.com/better/health/what-happens-your-body-brain-while-you-sleep-ncna805276

DiGiulio, S. (2017b, October 19). *How what you eat affects your sleep*. NBC News; NBC News. https://www.nbcnews.-com/better/health/how-what-you-eat-affects-how-you-sleep-ncna805256

Doheny, K. (2010, March 29). *Can't sleep? Adjust the temperature*. WebMD. https://www.webmd.com/sleep-disorders/features/cant-sleep-adjust-the-temperature

Dutta, S. (2016, March 7). *Causes of sleep deprivation*. News-Medical.net. https://www.news-medical.net/health/Causes-of-Sleep-Deprivation.aspx

Fletcher, J. (2019, February 12). *4-7-8 breathing: How it works, benefits, and uses* (T. Legg, Ed.). Www.medicalnewstoday.com. https://www.medicalnewstoday.com/articles/324417

Fry, A. (2021, June 3). *How noise can affect your sleep satisfaction* (N. Vyas, Ed.). Sleep Foundation. https://www.sleepfoundation.org/noise-and-sleep

Gotter, A. (2018, April 20). *What is the 4-7-8 breathing technique?* (T. Legg, Ed.). Healthline; Healthline Media. https://www.healthline.com/health/4-7-8-breathing

Havens, K. (2017, March 2). *How sleep position affects your spine.* Coastalorthoteam.com. https://www.-coastalorthoteam.com/blog/how-sleep-position-affects-your-spine

Mckinnen, G. (2020, November 13). *Avoid these bad sleep habits for a better night's rest.* Amerisleep.com. https://amerisleep.com/blog/bad-sleep-habits/

Moghim, R. (2020, February 21). *How your sleep posture impacts your health.* Colorado Pain Care. https://coloradopaincare.com/how-your-sleep-posture-impacts-your-health/

National Sleep Foundation. (2005). *Summary of findings: 2005 sleep in America poll.* https://www.sleepfoundation.org/wp-content/uploads/2018/10/2005_summary_of_findings.pdf?x16972

Newcomer, L. (2021, March 26). *LeBron James sleeps a lot. Here's why other athletes should too.* Mattress Clarity. https://www.mattressclarity.com/news/lebron-james-athletes-sleep/#:~:text=%E2%80%9CLe-bron%E2%80%A6%20has%20been%20quoted%20as

Nunez, K., & Lamoreux, K. (2020, July 20). *Why do we sleep? What happens during sleep?* Healthline. https://www.health-line.com/health/why-do-we-sleep

Pacheco, D. (2020, October 16). *Bedroom environment: What elements are important?* (A. Rehman, Ed.). Sleep Foundation. https://www.sleepfoundation.org/bedroom-environment

Pacheco, D. (2021, January 22). *Exercise and Sleep*. Sleep Foundation. https://www.sleepfoundation.org/physical-activity/exercise-and-sleep

Peri, C. (2010, February 18). *10 things to hate about sleep loss*. WebMD; WebMD. https://www.webmd.com/sleep-disorders/features/10-results-sleep-loss

Riccio, S. (2021, June 9). *How to choose the right pillow—2021 ultimate guide*. Sleepopolis. https://sleepopolis.-com/guides/right-pillow-how-to-choose/

Rosenberg, C. (2020, June 30). *What to do if your mind is racing before sleep*. Sleep Health Solutions. https://www.sleephealth-solutionsohio.com/blog/mind-racing-before-sleep/

Saber, S., Kianian, T., Navidia, A., & Aghamohamadi, F. (2017). Comparing the effects of aerobic and anaerobic exercise on sleep quality among male nonathlete students. *Nursing and Midwifery Studies, 6*(4), 168. https://doi.org/10.4103/nms.nms_56_17

Swiner, C. (2020, May 29). *What happens to your body when you sleep?* WebMD. https://www.webmd.com/sleep-disorders/ss/slideshow-sleep-body-effects

Vyas, N. (2020, August 14). *The best foods to help you sleep*. Sleep Foundation. https://www.sleepfoundation.org/nu-trition/food-and-drink-promote-good-nights-sleep

Watson, S., & Cherney, K. (2020, May 15). *11 effects of sleep deprivation on your body* (S. Sampson, Ed.). Healthline. https://www.healthline.com/health/sleep-deprivation/effects-on-body

Weiner, A. (2021, February 9). *The importance of the right bed sheets for a good night's sleep*. Elegant Strand. https://www.elegantstrand.com/blogs/news-1/the-importance-of-the-right-bed-sheets-for-a-good-night-s-sleep

Youngstedt, S. D., & Kline, C. E. (2006). Epidemiology of exercise and sleep. *Sleep and Biological Rhythms, 4*(3), 215–221. https://doi.org/10.1111/j.1479-8425.2006.00235.x

ABOUT THE AUTHOR

I used to work as an ordinary 9-to-5 employee just like most of the rest of the world. I was employed in a large corporation and was living paycheck to paycheck. Ultimately, I found myself mindlessly consenting to the rat race of life without having anything to show for it. After a while of participating in the same daily routine over and over again, I found that I needed to change things up. I needed a change of pace, and I asked my supervisor for permission to go on a vacation. Looking back now, I find it weird that I even needed to ask permission to do something as simple and as innocent as merely resting. That time away from work granted me the perspective to pursue my dreams of being an entrepreneur and forging my own path. I didn't want to subject myself to a timecard under the supervision of my company anymore. I wanted to control my own hours. In other words, I wanted to regain control of my own life.

Fast forward to today and I'm now a successful entrepreneur with various sources of income. This means that I have the flexibility and mobility to do whatever I want whenever I want. Part of what I'm doing is exploring my passion for writing. I've discovered that I've been blessed because of my renewed perspective on life and my approach to my career. I also know that there are many people out there who are unhappy with their lives in the same way that I was unhappy with mine. That's why I've committed myself to writing books just like this one to help people improve their lives based on the lessons that I had to learn the hard way.

All in all, I never realized just how badly my poor sleeping habits were affecting me. I had to discover the hard way that the way that I slept also directly impacted the way that I performed throughout the day. More than that, I realized that part of being able to succeed was knowing when to rest… and there's no better rest than sleep. I'm writing this book because I want to remind people that sleep is a vital component of success. I know that many out there are struggling to go to sleep at night, even when that shouldn't be the case. Hopefully, many of you will find comfort and solace in knowing that you aren't facing this challenge on your own and that many others are on the same boat as you. More than that, I hope that this book will provide you with the knowledge and perspective that you need to conquer your own sleep demons so that it will be easier for you to get your *zzz's* at night. Remember that success isn't all about working as hard as you can. It's also about picking your spots and knowing how to pace yourself. That's something that I discovered as I built my empire, and I'm hoping that by reading this book, you will also take this principle to heart.